Medicinal Plants in Industry
(Question Bank)

Medicinal Plants in Industry
(Question Bank)

A.V.S.S. SAMMBAMURTY

and

N.S. SUBRAHMANYAM

Readers, Department of Botany
Sri Venkateswara College
New Delhi-110021

CBS Publishers & Distributors Pvt. Ltd.

New Delhi • Bengaluru • Chennai • Kochi • Kolkata • Mumbai
Bhubaneswar • Hyderabad • Jharkhand • Nagpur • Patna • Pune • Uttarakhand • Dhaka

ISBN: 81-239-0665-X

First Edition: 2000
Reprint: 2007, 2020

Published by **Satish Kumar Jain** and produced by **Varun Jain** for **CBS Publishers & Distributors Pvt. Ltd.**,
4819/XI Prahlad Street, 24 Ansari Road, Daryaganj, New Delhi - 110002
delhi@cbspd.com, cbspubs@airtelmail.in • www.cbspd.com
Ph.: 23289259, 23266861, 23266867 • Fax: 011-23243014

Corporate Office: 204 FIE, Industrial Area, Patparganj, Delhi - 110 092
Ph: 49344934 • Fax: 011-49344935
E-mail: publishing@cbspd.com • publicity@cbspd.com

Branches:
- *Bengaluru:* 2975, 17th Cross, K.R. Road, Bansankari 2nd Stage, Bengaluru - 70 • Ph: +91-80-26771678/79 • Fax: +91-80-26771680
  E-mail: cbsbng@gmail.com, bangalore@cbspd.com
- *Chennai:* No. 7, Subbaraya Street, Shenoy Nagar, Chennai - 600030
  Ph: +91-44-26681266, 26680620 • Fax: +91-44-42032115
  E-mail: chennai@cbspd.com
- *Kochi:* Ashana House, 39/1904, A.M. Thomas Road, Valanjambalam, Ernakulum, Kochi • Ph: +91-484-4059061-65
  Fax: +91-484-4059065 • E-mail: cochin@cbspd.com
- *Kolkata:* 6-B, Ground Floor, Rameshwar Shaw Road, Kolkata - 700014
  Ph: +91-33-22891126/7/8 • E-mail: kolkata@cbspd.com
- *Mumbai:* 83-C, Dr. E. Moses Road, Worli, Mumbai - 400018
  Ph: +91-9833017933, 022-24902340/41 • E-mail: mumbai@cbspd.com

Representatives:

• Hyderabad: 0-9885175004	• Nagpur: 0-9021734563
• Patna: 0-9334159340	• Pune: 0-9623451994
• Jharkhand: 0-9811541605	• Uttarakhand: 0-9716462459

Printed at:
J.S. Offset Printers, Delhi (India)

PREFACE

How many people knew that *Taxus* and *Sassafras* are useful in the treatment of Cancer? Anti-Cancer antibiotics? About Ginseng? This book *Medicinal Plants in Industry* contains 1300 objective type Questions on current research in plant medicine - antibiotics, anti-cancer drugs, ginseng; alcoholic beverages, non-alcoholic beverages, gums and resins chemicals, oils from wild unexploited plants perfumes from plants; spices and condiments, tuber crops, herbs, tooth pastes, herbal cigarettes, dyes, tannins vegetables and fruits.

This work will be of great help to start small scale industries (for example see item nos. 436, 107 methi seeds, bari kateri seeds, contain diosgenin etc.;. These objective Questions are helpful to graduates, postgraduates and research scholars for obtaining recent information on economic uses of plants (Economic Botany).

The book will be greatly useful for students preparing for IAS, IFS, MBBS, ARS and for M.Sc students of Economic Botany, Ethnobotany and Plants and Human Welfare. The examples cited in the book cover wide range of plants of Industrial use especially in medicine and give answers for exploration of plant products by enthusiastic industrialists.

New Delhi   A.V.S.S. SAMMBAMURTY
1st Jan., 1999   N.S. SUBRAHMANYAM

CONTENTS

PHARMACOLOGY AND PHARMACOGNOSY OF MEDICINAL PLANTS

The discovery of plants for medicinal purposes to humans has a long antecedent history dating back to ancient civilizations. In medicine the product is important, apart from its other plant parts. For example, the medicinal principle will be found in their leaves, flowers, fruits, seeds, rhizomes, stems, roots, bark, flower buds, young leaves, and so on. Not only this, the timing of the active principle found in which part of the season, and also the time of the day are important, sometimes to get maximum effect of the medicine.

Hence, every part of the plant is to be tested for the medicinal compound and this branch of Pharmacy is called as *Pharmacognosy*. The chemical after it is extracted from the plant in its crude form has to be purified, crystallized and then marketed. This is the work of a pharmacist who is engaged in the preparation of medicines and then the industrialist utilizes these principles for releasing medicines into the market after certain legal procedures. Medicinal Botany offers great scope to industrialists, hitherto unexplored plants and introduce their products into the market for the benefit of the mankind.

For example, one company, called Neelchem Laboratories, in Nilgiris released a tea product called *DIATEA*, in which a plant product obtained from the leaves of *Gymnema sylvestre* (Asclepiadaceae) has been incorporated into ordinary tea for the benefit of the Diabetic persons. The leaves of this plant when chewed, temporarily destroy the capacity of tasting sugar, which is due to the presence of *Gymnemic acid* in the leaves. In this tea (DIATEA), 60% *Gymnema sylvestre* and 40% tea, *Camellia sinensis* are combined. This is a remarkable property, and if diabetic persons take this tea regularly in morning and evening or three times a day, can almost cure Diabetes.

Similarly, a private company from Kerala, CYBLE company

has been marketing a diabetic preparation under the trade name "Cogent db" in the form of tablets for diabetic persons. It consists of 9 plant products, viz.,

1. *Azadirachta indica*
2. *Phyllanthus emblica*
3. *Terminalia chebula*
4. *T. bellerica*
5. *Aconitum heterophyllum*
6. *Curcuma longa*
7. *Tribulus terrestris*
8. *Syzygium cumini*
9. *Rotula aquatica*

Like this, the search for new medicines in plants is a continued effort by industrialists. The old medicines give way for new medicines and chronic diseases like diabetes, cancer, asthma etc. can be cured in future. This book gives such hidden truths and interested persons can probe further to achieve their gigantic goals.

DEFINITIONS OF SOME TERMS IN MEDICAL BOTANY

Medical Botany — It is a branch that focuses on plants that injure, heal and nourish or alter the conscious mind.

Allergy — (Gr. *allos*, other; *ergon*, work). It is a condition of hypersensitivity of the body cells to specific substances resulting in various types of reactions.

Analeptic — The agent that excites and stimulates and causes generalised convulsions.

Angiodema — It is a condition of temporary swelling of skin associated with urticaria and erythema.

Ayurvedic Medicine — This is a branch of medicine based on the Hindu scriptures or Vedas. This type is considered indigenous in Indian system of medicine.

Compound System — The enzymatic system that is activated by antigen-antibody reactions and to activate and amplify the activity of successive components thus affecting chemotaxis, and bacteriolysis. The enzymatic system is composed of 9 separate components $C_1 - C_9$ and 11 serum proteins.

Depressant — These are the agents that reduce functional activity.

Dermatitis—This may be defined as a condition where inflammation of the skin is observed.

Diaphoretic—This is a condition which promotes perspiration.

Diplopia—This is referred when the vision is double.

Diuretic—The agent that increases urine flow is known as diuretic.

Edema—This is a condition where abnormal accumulation of fluid between the cells takes place.

Emetic—The agent that induces vomiting is known as emetic.

Epilepsy—This is a condition where disorder is characterized by severe muscular spasms.

Ergotism—This is a kind of disease showing spasms, cramps and various cerebrospinal disorders due to excessive use of ergot or of eating ergot containing grains.

Lathyrism—This is a kind of disease showing spastic paralegia, pain, hyperethesia and parathesia leading to death due to ingestion of seeds of a Leguminaceous species *Lathyrus*.

Myxedema—This is a kind of disorder which is hypothyroid induced and is characterized by dry waxy skin due to mucin deposits.

Neuroleptic—This is tranquilizing agent, generally without hypnotic effect and is generally observed as psychomotor activity.

Peristalsis—It is an action where rhythmatic contraction and relaxation along the intestine promoting movement of contents.

Pharmacognosy—The study of natural drugs and their natural constituents is known as pharmacognosy.

Photodermatitis—This is an inflammation of skin resulting from activation by light of chemicals on the skin.

Phytohemagglutinin (PHA)—It is a plant product, called mitogenic lectin, that agglutinates erythrocytes and stimulates thymus-derived lymphocytes.

Pyretic—It is referred to as kind of fever.

Rheumatic Fever—This is a kind of fever due to inflammation of heart fibrous tissue leading to scarring of heart valves and the joints; occurs as an immunological sequel to *Streptococcus pyrogens* infection elsewhere.

Schizophrenia—This is a mental disease that involves the disorganization of personality and characterized by delusions, hallucinations, abnormal behaviour and retreat from reality.

Sedative—It is an agent used to relieve tension and anxiety.

Synesthesia—It is a condition in which a stimulus of one sense is perceived as sensation of a different sense.

Thrush—It is due to infection by *Candida sp.* (Fungi Imperfecti) of oral mucous membranes, usually in childhood.

Toxicomania—This is referred to periodic or chronic state of intoxication as a result of repeated use of a drug harmful to the individual or society.

Unani Medicine—This is a branch of medical are based on traditional medical system found in the Muslim World.

Wheal and flare—The immediate response to histamine release or other minor nonpenetrating injury to the skin is known as wheal and flare. This is followed by wheal or edema radiating from the line of injury. It is considered as a characteristic skin lesion of immediate hypersensitivity.

ALLERGEN

The substances that are capable of inducing an allergic response are known as allergens. The allergic response is observed by the hypersensitivity of body cells to various types of reactions.

Generally every living organism can produce an immune system and can protect the body from disease. During the protection process, a system is developed by which many mechanisms are evolved which increase the efficiency of recognition and elimination of foreign proteins (antigens). The present concept of antigen relates that the reticuloendothelial system can recognise an antigen after contact and results in the production of immunoreactive cells (due to immune response) and modified serum globulins (immunoglobulins) which can eliminate the specific antigen from the body. These cells persist as immune response cells that can recognise subsequent antigens by contact.

The development of immunoglobins (the antibodies) is related to hypersensitivity. This may cause hay fever, asthma and anaphylactic shock. The antibody is formed due to the contact of allergen locally within plasma cells embedded in the mucosa of target areas of the nasopharynx, gastrointestinal tracts and respiratory tracts. The allergen diffuses into the tissue fluid, and the antibody attaches to the basophils and platelets. Then the allergen binds to this cell bound reagin (reaginic antibody). The attachment triggers the release of histamine, kinins, serotonin and other vasoactive substances. Now the allergic symptoms in the form of vasodilation, bronchospasm and increased nasal secretion is produced.

The allergic symptom can be reduced by introducing small amounts of the allergen or white cell response. The cell response binds the allergen and prevents reagin-allergen complexes. The allergen is due to spore or pollen (seasonal allergy), and the preventive method may be attempted preseasonally, ensuring that blocking antibodies are at their highest during provocative period.

AEROALLERGENS

The wind borne inciting allergens are known aeroallergens. These allergens produce allergic rhinitis, bronchial asthma and hyper- sensitivity pneumonitis.

1. Allergic rhinitis

The wind pollinated plants elicit symptoms of allergic rhinitis, or hay fever. The symptoms are—profuse watery nasal discharge, sneezing, irritated and watery eyes and headache. The spores from fungi and even certain algae are responsible for such symptoms. The grass pollens are aeroallergens..

The plants that are pollinated through animals induce allergic rhinits. The attractive roses frequently used to lead to sensitization through inhalation of pollen and the term rose fever is used to describe plant associated rhinitis.

2. Asthma

If a specific allergen is inhalated, the attacks of bronchial asthma is observed. This is hypersensitive respiratory ailment caused by exposure of the respiratory epithelium to allergens. Histamins and serotonin are involved in the symptoms e.g. asthmatic wheezing, viscid bronchial secretion etc. This is due to inhalation of aerollergens such as spores, feathers and animal tenders.

3. Hypersensitivity pneumonitis

Persons of specific profession like farmers, cheeseworkers, brewers etc. are often associated with another kind of allergic respiratory condition known as hypersensitivity pneumonitis. The symptoms are—watery eyes, sneezing, an irritating sensation in the nasal passages, soreness of the throat and dry cough.

The inciting allergen can be detected by several provocative tests of skin. The introduction of dilute concentration of allergen into the skin by intradermal injection is a frequently employed method. If a specific reaginic antibody is present in the skin, the characteristic erythema of cutaneous anaphylaxis reactions appear within few minutes. Recently Radio Allergo Sorbent Test (RAST) on binding antibody to antigen in a system containing radio labelled antibody, Passive Leukocyte Sensitizing Test (PLS) have been used.

Therapy

The seeds of *Ammi visnaga* (family Apiaceae) yield a new compound called cromolyn sodium. This compound is believed to affect the release of vasoactive substances and act to prevent the asthma. The leaves of *Tylophora indica* (family Asclepiadaceae) is claimed to relieve moderate to complete action of nasobronchial allergic symptoms.

There are three drugs that are used to control asthmatic attacks. They are epinephrine (adrenalin) and its congeners administered by aerosal, the methylxanthines administered intravenously for chronic asthma and steroids (cortisone) for severe and intractable states.

PLANTS CAUSING ALLERGY

Angiosperms

Aceraceae	—	*Acer*
Arecaceae	—	*Phoenix*
Asteraceae	—	*Arubrosea, Taraxacum*
Betulaceae	—	*Alnus, Betula*
Brassicaceae	—	*Sinapsis*
Cyperaceae	—	*Carex*
Euphorbiaceae	—	*Mercurialis*
Fabaceae	—	*Acacia*
Fagaceae	—	*Fagus, Quercus*
Juncaceae	—	*Juncus*
Moraceae	—	*Morus*
Myrtaceae	—	*Eucalyptus*
Polygonaceae	—	*Rheum, Rumex*
Ranunculaceae	—	*Ranunculus*
Scrophulariaceae	—	*Verbascum*
Typhaceae	—	*Typha*
Tiliaceae	—	*Tilia*
Urticaceae	—	*Urtica*

Gymnosperms

Thuja, Pinus, Juniperus, Ginkgo

Algae

Chlorella

Fungi

Rhizopus, Erysiphe, Puccinia, Candida, Alternaria, Monilia, Phoma.

IRRITANT ALLERGENIC PLANTS

Araceae
  Alocasia, Arum, Colocasia
Brassicaceae
  Brassica
Euphorbiaceae
  Jatropha
Fabaceae
  Acacia, Mucuna
Lamiaceae
  Leonotis
Liliaceae
  Alium
Moraceae
  Cecropia, Maclura
Poaceae
  Bambusa
Solanaceae
  Capscicum
Sterculiaceae
  Sterculia
Urticaceae
  Fleurya, Laportea

PHOTOSENSITIZING ALLERGENIC PLANTS

Apiaceae	—	*Ammi majus*
		Anethum graveolens
		Apium graveolens
Brassicaceae	—	*Brassica sp.*
Moraceae	—	*Ficus carica*
Ranunculaceae	—	*Ranunculus sp.*
Rosaceae	—	*Agrimonia eupatoria*
Rutaceae	—	*Dictamnus albus*
		Ruta graveolens

SKIN ALLERGENS OF PLANT ORIGIN

Name	Active Principles	Chemical nature
Apiaceae		
Apium sp.	Limonene	Terpenes
Rutaceae		
Citrus sp.	"	"
Lamiaceae		
Mentha spicata	Phellandrene	"
Lauraceae		
Cinnamomum sp.	"	"
Geraniaceae		
Pelargonium sp.	Geraniol	Alcohol
Rosaceae		
Rosa	Citronellol	"
Zingiberaceae		
Elettaria		
Cardamomum	Borneal	"
Poaceae		
Cymbopogon	Citral	Aldehyde
Asteraceae		
Blumea	Camphore	Ketones

CANCER PROHIBITING DRUGS

Among the diseases of man, cancer is most feared and baffling. There are several hundred different types of cancer and these are associated with rapid and uncontrolled formation of abnormal cells in the body. The abnormal cells mass together to form a growth or proliferate individually throughout the body, they serve no useful function to the body, furthermore the cells may interfere with the function of the organ or tissue in which they are found. The cells may invade the neighbouring tissues and in metastasis they enter the blood stream. Malignant cells also spread throughout the body through lymphatic vessels.

The plant products may cause this type of development of abnormal cells. The excessive use of snuff from *Nicotiana tabacum* causes the appearance of fatal malignant polyps of the nose. Tannin-rich plants are the source of incidence of nasal cancer.

The workers of leather industry and wood industry are prone to neoplasia. The plant *Annona muricata* is rich in tannin and causes this type of disease. The black tea has been noted as very rich in tannins. These potentially dangerous compounds are rendered insoluble by milk, for the casein of milk fixes the tannin and prevents its action on the mucous membrane of the mouth.

Some members of the family Asteraceae (e.g. *Senecio*), Boraginaceae (e.g. *Heliotropium*) and Fabaceae (e.g. *Crotalaria*) contain pyrrolizidine alkaloids that are known to be hepato-carcinogenic. The dried ground leaves and stem of *Heliotropium supinum* (Boraginaceae) have been found in rats to cause pancreatic tumours. The South African *Senecio longilobus* (Asteraceae) form a high proportion of hepatic tumours.

The chewing of three distinct quids—betel, which includes the seeds of *Areca'* leaf of *Piper*, lime and various additions of tobacco, oil of cotton seeds and cocoa (*Erythroxylon coca*) have alkaloids and cause oral cancer.

The alkaloids are released by the addition of lime and thus hastening the physiological effects by damaging the oral mucous membrane. Certain metabolites from molds and bacteria are potential carcinogens. *Clavieps purpurea* develops multiple fibormas in the ears of rat. *Pencillium islandicum* is linked with hepatotoxic and hepatomalignant substances. *Fusarium griseofulvin* is associated treatment of human skin infection. A *spergillus flavus*, A. *parasiticus* contain aflatoxin. Aflatoxin and mycotoxin poisoning is fatal to children. *Agaricus bisporus*, the edible mushroom has been found to possess ethionine, a synthetic carcinogen which is a metabolite of common gut bacterium, *Escherischia coli*. Seaweeds (members of algal group) contain carrageenan which induces sarcomas at the site of infections.

Cycas circinalis seeds and roots contain cycasin, *Cycas revoluta* contains neocycasin, species of *Macrozamia* contain *macrozamin*. All are highly toxic and are related to nitrosamines.

Cancer Chemotherapeutic Drugs of Plant Origin

Species	Active compound (of Drugs)	Toxicity
Vinca roseus	Vinblastine (drug Velban) Vincristine sulfate (drug Oncovin)	Local irritant stomatitis, Paralytic ileus
Streptomyces parvullus	Dactinomycin (actinomycin D)	Stomatitis, oral ulcers
Streptomyces verticillatus	Bleomycin sulfate	Pulmonary fibrosis Edema of hand
Streptomyces peucetius	Adriamycin	Cardiotoxicity Stomatitis

Cancer Chematherapeutic Drugs of Higher plants

Catharanthus roseus	Apocynaceae — Vinblastine sulfate
Podophyllum emodi	— Berberidaceae — 4' — Demethylepi-podophyllotoxin
Cephaelis ipecacuanha	— Rubiaceae — Emetine
Eupatorium cuneifolium	— Asteraceae — Eupacunin
Senecio triangularis	— Asteraceae — Senecionine

REMEDIAL PLANTS

Croton macrostachys	— Euphorbiaceae — Crotepoxide
Crotalaria assamica	— Fabaceae — Monocrotaline
Sanguinaria canadensis	— Papaveraceae — Sanguinarine
Rumex hymenosepalus	— Polygonaceae — Leucopelargonidin
Thalictrum minum	— Ranunculaceae

Solanum dulcamara
— Thalidasine
— Solanaceae
— β-solamarine

List of stimulative drugs

Disease	Drugs of plant origin
Rheumatoid arthritis	*Aralia racemosa* — root
Aching backs	*Harnamelis virginiana* — boiled leaves and a stem.
Chronic rheumatism	*Phytolacca americana*-fruit
Convulsions, Epilepsy	*Datura stramonium* seed extract *Heracleum lanatum*
Depressants and Sedative	*Cypirpedium sp.* nerve sedative *Passiflora incarnata* nerve sedative *Veleriana officinalis* nerve sedative.
Fevers	*Cornus florida* — flower *Oldenladia corymbosa* *Myrica cerifera*
Headaches	*Arisaema atrorubens* — dried roots
Insomnia	*Solanum americanum* — leaves in large quantity
Mental disease	*Canthium glabriflorum* — root *Capparis tomentosum* — leaf and bark
Neuralgia	*Caesalpinia dignya, Tinospora cordifolia*

Cardiac drugs of plant origin

Plants	Active ingredient
Apocynum cannabinum — roots (Apocynaceae)	Cymarin
Strophanthus gratus-seeds (Apocyneaceae)	Ovabain

(Contd.)

Nerium oleander — leaf (Apocynaceae)	Oleandrin
Selenicerus grandiflorus — Stems (Cactaceae)	Acetyldigitoxin
Digitalis lanata — leaves (Scrophulariaceae)	Digitoxin
Adonis vernalis-rhizome and roots —Ranunculaceae	Admonitory
Convallaria majalis — rhizome (Liliaceae)	Convallatoxin

Vasopressure property of some plants

Plant	Alkaloid
Ephedra sinica Ephedra equisetina (whole plant)	Ephedrin
Phoradendron flaveuscous — leaves	Tyramine
Arthrophytum leptocladum	Dipterin
Acacia sp.	Tryptamine
Citrus sp. (fruit)	Herperidin
Eucalyptus macrorhynchia	Rutin
Claviceps purpurea	Ergonovine

URINARY PROBLEMS AND ITS THERAPY

There are some disturbances in urinary tract that the flow of urine is not normal. This condition is counteracted by some chemical that induce a net loss of fluid from the body of the urinary tracts. these chemicals are known as diuretic and it influences the flow of urine.

The nature of diuretic property is observed in many plant

species, they are:

  (a) *Equisetum arvense* (plant)—Pteridophyte
  (b) *Coffea arabica* (fruit)—Rubiaceae
  (c) *Withania somnifera* (root)—Solanaceae
  (d) *Abutilon indicum* (root)—Malvaceae
  (e) *Clematis biondtana* (plant)—Ranunculaceae
  (f) *Boerhaavia diffusa* (plant)—Nyctaginaceae
  (g) *Urtica dioica* (plant)—Urticaceae
  (h) *Costus spicatus* (sap)—Zingiberaceae
  (i) *Spiranthes diuretica* (plant)—Orchidaceae

The diverse ailments of urinary system include renal and bladder stones and infections of various kinds. The following plants are used as remedies for the disorders:

  (a) *Ephedra nevadensis*—seeds are served to alleviate urogenital diseases.

  (b) *Asimina reticulata* (Annonaceae)—flowers are used as hot drink to relieve the kidney trouble.

  (c) *Eryngium campestre* (Apiaceae)—root extracts are used against diseases of bladder and uterine irritation.

  (d) *Eupatorium purpureum* (Asteraceae)—rhizomes are used in the treatment of bladder stones. The roots of *Caesalpinia nuga* (Fabaceae) are used for gravel and stones in the bladder.

  (e) *Solanum mammosum* (Solanaceae)—leaf decoctions are valued for ailments of the bladder and kidney. *Arundo kakao*(Poaceae) stems have been employed for kidney ailments.

Genital problems and therapy

There are some compounds that block the production of female sex hormone and thus the ovulation process is delayed. This is done for the purpose of birth control. The discovery of semisynthetic steroids opened the way of such processes. The compounds are generally designated as contraceptive and may be used orally. The contraceptive contains estrogen and progestin, which supress the pituitary hormone through negative feedback and to stimulate the endometrium of the uterus initiating a menstrual cycle. The pituitary production of ovary influencing hormone is suppressed signalling the cessation of further ovary function.

In old days, there are many folk medicines that are used as oral contraceptives. The unripe spadix of *Urospatha antisylleptica*

(Araceae) and root of *Veratrum californicum* (Liliaceae) are taken daily for 3 weeks for sterility.

There are some compounds that stimulate uterine and hastening the rapidity of labor. These compounds are known as oxytocic agents. Before the clinical use of these agents, the medievel midwife used to give rye grains contaminated with ergot (fungus) to women in labor. Their observation includes speeder births and recoveries with far less of blood. The rye grains contaminated with fungus ergot (*Claviceps purpurea*) bear two alkaloids ergonovine and methylergonovine. These compounds are used after parturition to produce firm uterine contractions and to decrease postpartum uterine bleeding. Strong uterine contractions and short delivery time are normally observed with *Oldenlandia offinis* (Rubiaceae) stem and leaf is drunk before actual childbirth. Other plant compounds that are used as a drug to aid childbirth are: (a) *Diascorea villous* (Diascoreaceae)-rihzomes and roots are taken with hot water in difficult cases of childbirth. (b) *Regimen philadelphians* (Astrachan)-leaves and flowering tops are used. (c) *Trillium grandiflorum* (Liliaceae)-roots are employed to facilitate parturition. (d) *Gossypium sp.* (Malacca)-roots are taken as tea to ease labour. (e) *Petulant bumpily* (Petulance)-a postparturition tonic was prepared from Cones". (f) *Caesalpinia nougat* Caesalpiniaceae powdered leaves employed as a uterine tonic following childbirth. (g) *Fuchsia excortica* (Onagraceae)-extracts arrest haemorrhage after childbirth. Some plant products are used for effective fertility control as abortifacients. They are: (a) *Chrysanthemum parthenon* (Astrachan)-dried flowers have been used to induce abortion. (b) *Chelators paniculata* (Celastraceae)-bark extract is used to terminate pregnancy. (c) *Urginea pure* (Liliaceae)-bark decoction is used to induce abortion. (d) *Avicennia marina* (Verbenaceae)-the aromatic bitter juice is abortive.

STIMULANTS OF SEXUAL DESIRE (Aphrodisiacs) There are some plants that possess volatile oil, have nutritive value and affect neuromuscular system. These properties produce effect on sexual desire and act as a sexual stimulant or tonic. An alkaloid (Yohimbine) derived from *Coronaches johimbe*(Rubiaceae) has been employed as sexual stimulant drug and commercially it is available as johimbine hydrochloride combined with methyl testosterone and nux-vomica (seeds of *Strychnine*).

(a) *Hydrophobia ausculate* (Acanthaceae)-seeds are used as asphrodisiacs.

(b) *Heracleum wallichii* (Apiaceae) — roots are employed to prepare a tonic that acts on nervous system and stimulate sexual desire.

(c) *Holarrhena antidysentrica* (Apocynaceae) seeds are used as tonic.

(d) *Aristolochia indicia* (Aristolochiaceae) — rhizomes are stimulants and helpful for impotence.

(e) *Sphaeranthus indicus* (Asteraceae) — root, powerful stimulating agent.

(f) *Spearmints indices* (Astrachan) — seed

(g) *Tricholopsis globerimum* (Asteraceae) — whole plant

(h) *Cannabis indica* (Cannabinaceae) — dried pistillate flower formerly used as powerful aphrodisiacs but prolonged use may lead to impotence.

(i) *Butea monosperma* (Fabaceae) — flower and leaf

(j) *Crocus sativus* (Iridaceae) — dried stigmas

(k) *Eulophia campestris* (Orchidaceae) — rhizome

(l) *Orchis latifolia* (Orchidaceae) — tuber, valuable aphrodisiac

(m) *Brunfelsia grandiflora* (Solanaceae) — root

(n) *Mandragora officinarum* (Solanaceae) — root

(o) *Withania somnifera* (Solanaceae) — root

(p) *Alpinia galange* (Zingiberaceae) — rhizome

Some depressive drugs like narcotics, barbiturates, tranquilizers are capable of inhibiting sexual desire (i.e. they are anaphrodisiacs). Cyproterone acetate is a drug used in Great Britain in treating rapists and other convicted of sex crimes. This drug lowers the male sex drive by blocking the function of testosterone. *Vitex agnuscastus* (Verbenaceae) has been known to possess this property and its reference was cited in folk medicine. Seeds of *Nymphaea alba* (Nymphaeaceae) has been considered effective in lowering sexual desire.

There are diseases in sexual parts in both male and female due to some transmittable microbes through infected venereal contact to genitals and through formites to vulvovagina of prepubertal girls. In the male, urethritis occurs through invasion of the epithelium of the anterior urethra and urethral glands. In female similar complication may occur and the infection spreads from the urethra and cervix to uterus, Fallopian tubes and ovarian surfaces. The disease is gonorrhea. The following plant extracts are used to treat the disease.

(a) *Cassia surratensis* (Caesalpiniaceae) — root decoction
(b) *Paradaniella oliveri* (Fabaceae) — root decoction
(c) *Arctium lappa* (Asteraceae) — root
(d) *Liatris spicata* (Asteraceae) — plant
(e) *Solanum agrarium* (Solanaceae) — leaf decoction
(f) *Galium ambrosum* (Rubiaceae) — plant
(g) *Thapsia montana* (Apiaceae) — shrub decoction.

Syphilis is another kind of venereal disease. The disease is a continuous and leads to a hard black painless chancre, eruptions and autoimmune gummosis and cardiovascular and nerve damage. Infection in uterous may develop congenital malformations particularly of the teeth and bones.

The plant extracts used to treat the disease are:

(a) *Smilax medica* (Liliaceae) — root
(b) *Corydalis gavaniana* (Papaveraceae) — root
(c) *Cayaponia espelina* (Cucurbitaceae) —.root
(d) *Urena caracasana* (Urticaceae) — whole plant
(e) *Tabernaemontana corymbosa* (Apocynaceae) — bark decoction

Penicillin is used in all stages of syphilis treatment. Surveilliance through blood testing is used in detection and cure of syphills.

There are other types of venereal diseases

(a) *Chancroid* — is characterised by one or more painful genital ulcerations. This infection is treated with erythronycine and tetracyline.

(b) *Lymphogranuloma nonereum* — infection with *Chlamydia* sp. lymphadenitis and draining buboes are common. This infection is treated with sulfa drugs, erythromycine and tetracycline.

(c) *Granuloma inguinale*-is characterised by ulcerogranulomalous lesions involving the skin and mucosa of the genital and inguinal areas. This disease is caused by the infection of *Donovania granulomatis* and the infection can be treated with erythromycine and tetracycline.

PSYCHOACTIVE PLANTS

The number of plant products that influence the nervous system are many and particular groups that act on central nervous system are treated as psychoactive plants. The range of effect is wide for these plants and they are:

Stimulants — which excite and enhance psychomotor activity

Hallucinogens — which induce dream like state

Depressants — which reduce mental and physical performance.

Lists of some Hallucinogenic compounds of plant origin

S. No.	Plant	Vernacular Name	Active Hallucinogenic Principle
1.	*Claviceps purpurea* (Fungi)	Ergot	D-Lysergic acid
2.	*Amanita muscaria* (Fungi)	Fly agaric	Ibotenic acid, muscimol
3.	*Myristica fragrans* (Myristicaceae)	Nutemeg and mace	Nonnsitrogenous phenylpropanes
4.	*Lophophora williamsii* (Cactaceae)	Peyote	β-phenylethylamines
5.	*Cannabis sativa* (Cannabinaceae)	Marihuana, Hemp, Bhang	Nonnitrogenous tetrahydrocannabianal
6.	*Sophora secundiflora* (Fabaceae)	Mescal bean	Cytisine
7.	*Tabemanthe iboga* (Apocynaceae)	Iboga	Ibogaine

(Contd.)

8. *Atropa belladona* (Solanaceae)	Belladona	Hyoscyamine, Scopolamine
9. *Hyoscymus niger* (Solanaceae)	Henbane	Hyoscyamine
10. *Mandragora officinarum* (Solanaceae)	Mandrake	Hyoscyamine
11. *Ipomoea violacea* (Convolvulaceae)	Morining glory	Dtysergic acid
12. *Acorus calamus* (Araceae)	Sweet flag	Asarone

The knowledge of natural products established a separate branch of plant science known as *pharmacognosy*. The term is derived from two Greek words-*pharmakon*, the drug and *gnosis*-the knowledge. In 1815 C.A. Seydler, a medical student in Germany introduced this term. In this knowledge, the application of various scientific disciplines was employed and the knowledge of drug from every point of view was the main object of this study. Modern aspects of this branch include not only the crude plant products but also their natural derivatives. *Cinchona* bark and its purified alkaloid quinine (alkaloid) is the part of the subject matter of pharmacognosy.

Pharmacology — is defined as an applied science that deals with the study of action of drugs.

Crude Drug — is defined as the plant or animal drugs consisting of natural substances that have undergone only the processes of collection and drying.

Organoleptic Evaluation — refers to evaluation by means of the organs of sense. Literally it means impression on the organs.

Active Constituents — It is referred to the chemical entities that are responsible for the therapeutic effect. Pharmaceutically active constituents may cause precipitation or other chemical changes in medicinal preparation. Pharmacologically active constituents may be either single chemical substances or mixtures of principles and are responsible for the therapeutic activity of the drug. Cinchotanic acid is a pharmaceutically active constituents. Sugars, starches, glycosides, or mixtures of fixed oils, resins etc. are pharmacologically active constituents.

Drug Biosynthesis — The study of the biochemical pathway of drug constituents leading to the information of secondary constituents used as drugs is known as drug biosynthesis.

Allergy — It is defined as describing a changed or altered reaction due to antigenic substances capable of sensitizing body.

Adulteration — Mixing inferior and spurious ingredients for commercial purposes.

COMMERCIAL DRUGS

The drugs of commercial origin are referred as commercial drugs. These drugs generally are trade products with some geographic name. This indicates the region in which they are collected but not necessarily reflect the area where the plant grows. For example, the commercial gum (*Acacia senegal*) now comes from trees cultivated in Sudan, though the plant is abundant in Senegal. Similarly, the Peru balsam does not come from Peru but is produced in E1 Salvador. Thus the commercial origin may change in course of time.

Preparation of commercial drug — As pharmacognosy embraces the knowledge of history, distribution, cultivation of economic important plants, the following steps are used for the preparation of drugs of commercial market.

I. Collection—The collection of plant material must be done when the part of the plant that constitutes the drug is highest in its content of active principles and when the material will dry to give the maximum quality and appearance.

The collection must be done from cultivated plants. This ensures a true natural source and a reliable product. Many drugs are collected from wild plants. In this case the collectors should be serious and careful to avoid non-therapeutic plants.

II. Harvesting—The harvesting process is most important step as it is related to the nature and quantity of constituents. Quite natural, the mode of harvesting varies with each drug produced. Harvesting may be done by hand or by mechanical devices. As the cost of labour is increasing day by day, the use of mechanical devices is economic and now widely used. The time of harvesting should be noted as in case of roots and underground parts when the vegetative portion dies, the bark should be removed in the spring and it is done by hand stripping. The leaves should be harvested in its full growing phase. It is end of March to Ist week of October and it is done by hand.

III. Drying — This process is done to ensure good keeping qualities and action of enzymes. Drying fixes the constituents, facilitates grinding and milling and converts the drug into a more convenient form of commercial handling. It involves control of temperature and regulation of air flow. The plant material can be dried either by the sun or by the use of artificial heat.

IV. Garbling — This is the last step in preparation of drug. In this step, removal of extraneous matter dirt and added adulterants, is done.

V. Packaging — The drug material so far garbled, should be kept in a good package that provides ample protection and gives economy of space. Leaves and herbaceous material is usually baled with power balers into a solid compact mass and is then sewn into burlap cover. Moisture proof cans should be used for plant material that are likely to deteriorate from absorbed moisture.

VI. Storage—This step ensures the maintainance of high degree of quality of the drug. The storage must be done in fire proof steel, concrete or brick built houses. The warehouses should be built in such a manner that there is no possibility of causing undesirable changes in constituents as light affects the drug and oxygen increases the oxidation of the constituents of drug. Excessive moisture facilitates fungal growth. Therefore. the warehouse should be cool, dark and well ventilated with dry air.

VII. Protection and preservation — Protection means the action against the attack of insects or other microorganisms. There are number of methods for the protection-use of high temperature (65°C), the use of fumigation and the use of chemicals like methyl bromide.

Some important members of underground parts containing drugs.

Name	Family importance	Medicinal
1. *Dryopteris filix-mas*	Polypdiaceae (pteridophyte)	Toxic on tape worms
2. *Valeriana officinalis*	Velerianaceae	Carminative
3. *Veratrum album*	Liliaceae	Emetic and purgative
4. *Rheum pulmatum*	Polygonaceae	Mild laxative and intestinal astrigent
5. *Ferula sumbul*	Umbelliferae	Antispasmodic
6. *Arnica montana*	Compositae	Prevents swelling
7. *Zingiber officinalis*	Zinziberaceae	Carminative
8. *Colchicum autumnale*	Liliaceae	Pain reliever

IMPORTANT MEDICINAL PLANTS, THEIR CONSTITUENTS AND USES

1. *Allium sativum* (Liliaceae)
   GARLIC
   A bulbous perennial growing to 30 cm - 1 m (1-3 ft), with pale pink or green-white flowers.

   Key Constituents:
   Volatile oil (alliin, allinase, allicin)
   Scordinins
   Selenium
   Vitamins A,B,C and E

   Key Actions:
   Antibiotic
   Expectorant
   Increase sweating
   Lowers blood pressure
   Reduces blood clotting
   Anti-diabetic
   Expels worms

2. *Aloe vera syn. A. barbadensis* (Liliaceae)
   ALOE VERA, ALOES
   A perennial with succulent leaves 60 cm (2 ft) long and a spike
   of yellow or orange flowers.

   Key Constituents:
   Anthraquinones (aloin, aloe-emodin)
   Resins
   Tannins
   Polysaccharides
   Aloectin B

   Key Actions:
   Heals wounds
   Emollient
   Stimulates secretions of bile
   Laxative

3. *Alpinia officinarum* (Zingiberaceae)
   GALANGAL (HINDI), GAO LIANG (CHINESE)
   A perennial aromatic plant growing to 2 m (6 ft), with white,
   redlipped flowers and lance-shaped leaves.

   Key constituents:
   Volatile oil (about 1%) containing alpha-pinence, cineole,
   linalool.
   Sesquiterpene lactones (galangol, galangin)
   Key Actions:
   Warming digestive tonic
   Stimulant
   Carminative
   Prevents vomiting
   Antifungal

4. *Ammi visnaga syn. Daucus visnaga* (Umbelliferace)
   VISNAGA, KHELLA
   An erect annual growing to 1m (3 ft.) with leaves divided into
   wisps and clusters of small white flowers.
   Key constituents:
   Khellin (1%)
   Visnagin

Khellol glycoside
Volatile oil (0.2%)
Flavonoids
Sterols
Key actions:
Antispasmodic
Anti-asthmatic
Relaxant

5. *Angelica sinensis* (Umbelliferae)
   CHINESE ANGELICA, DAND CUT (CHINESE)
   A stout,erect perennial growing to 2m, with large bright given
   leaves and hollow stems.

   Key Constituents:
   Coumarins
   Volatile oil (butylidine phthalide, ligustilide, sesqiter-penes,
   carvacrol)
   Vitamin B_{12}
   Beta-sitosterol

   Key Actions:
   Tonic
   Blood tonic
   Antispasmodic
   Sedative
   Promotes menstrual flow

6. *Apium graveolens* (Umbelliferace)
   CELERY, SMALLAGE
   A biennial with a ridged shiny stem, glossy leaves and small
   flowers, growing to about 50 cm (20 in).

   Key constituents:
   Volatile oil (1.5-3%) containing limonene (60-70%), phthalides
   and beta-selinene.
   Coumarins
   Furancomarins (bergapten)
   Furanoids (aplin)

Key actions:
Antirhenmatic
Carminative
Antispasmodic
Diuretic
Lowers blood pressure
Urinary antiseptic

7. *Arctium lappa* (Compositae)
   BURDOCK, NIU BANG ZI (Chinese)
   A biennial, with stems that grow to 1.5 m, reddish purple
   flowerheads and hooked bracts.

   Key Constituents:
   Bitter glycosides (arctiopicrin)
   Flavonoids (arctin)
   Tannins
   Polyacetylenes
   Volatile oil
   Inulin (up to 45%)
   Sesquiterpenes

   Key Actions:
   Cleansing
   Mild diuretic
   Antibiotic
   Antiseptic

8. *Artemisia absinthium* (Compositae)
   WORMWOOD
   A perennial reaching 1 m, with grey-green stems and feathery
   leaves, both covered in fine hairs.

   Key Constituents:
   Volatile oil containing sesquiterpene lactones (artabsin,
   anabsinthin); thujone; azulenea.
   Flavonoids
   Phenolic acids
   Lignans

Key Action:
Aromatic bitter
Stimulates secretion of bile
Anti-inflammatory
Eliminates worms
Eases stomach pain
Mild antidepressant

9. *Artemisia annua* (Compositae)
QING HAO, CHINESE WORMWOOD
A perennial growing to about 1 m, with green feathery leaves covered in fine hairs.

Key Consitituents:
Volatile oil (abrotamine, beta-bourbonene)
Sesquiterpene lactone (artemisinin)
Vitamin A

Key Actions:
Bitter
Reduces fever
Antimalarial
Antibiotic

10. *Astragalus membranaceus* (Leguminosae)
ASTRAGALUS, MILK VETCH, HUANG QI (CHINESE)
A perennial growing to 40 cm, with hairy stems and leaves divided into 12-18 pairs of leaflets.

Key Constituents:
Asparagine
Calcyosin
Formononetin
Astragalo sides
Kumatakenin
Sterols

Key Actions:
Adaptogenic
Immune stimulant
Diuretic

Vasodiclator
Antiviral

11. *Atropa belladonna* (Solanaceae)
DEALLY NIGHTSHADE, BELLADONNA
A perennial with large leaves and black berries, growing to
1.5 m.

Key Constituents:
Tropane alkaloids (up to 0.%), including hyoscyamine and
atropine.
Flavonoids
Coumarins
Volatile bases (nicotinc)

Key Actions:
Smooth muscle antispasmodic
Narcotic
Reduces sweating
Sedative

12. *Barosma betulina* (Rutaceae)
BUCHU
A bushy shrub growing to 2 m, with stemless, slightly leathery
leaves dotted with oil glands.

Key Constituents:
Volatile oil (1.5-2.5%), including pulegone, menthone,
diosphenol.
Sulphur compounds
Flavonoids (diosmin, rutin)
Mucilage

Key Actions:
Urinary antiseptic
Diuretic
Stimulant
Uterine stimulant

13. *Bupleurum Chinese* syn. *B. scorzoneraefolium* (Umbelliferae)
BUPLEURUM,HARE'S EAR ROOT< CHAT HU (CHINESE)
A perennial growing to 1 m high, with sickl-shaped
leaves and clusters of small yellow flowers.

Key Constituents:
Bupleurumol
Triterpenold saponins-saikosides (saikonina)
Flavonoids (rutin)

Key Actions:
protects liver
Anti-inflammatory
Tonic
Antiviral

14. *Calendula officinalis* (Compositae)
MARIGOLD, POT MARIGOLD
An annual growing to 60 cm, with vivid orange flower-heads
similar in structure to daisies.

Key Constituents:
Triterpenes
Resins
Bitter glycosides
Volatile oil
Sterols Flavonoids
Mucilage
Caratenes

Key actions:
Anti-inflammatory
Relieves muscle spasms
Astringent
Prevents haemorrhaging
Heals wounds
Antiseptic
Detoxifying
Mildly oestrogenic

15. *Capsicum frutescens* (Solanaceae)
    CAYENNE, CHILLI
    A perennial, spiky shrub growing to 1 m, with scarletred conical fruits with seeds.

    Key constituents:
    Capsaicin (0.1-1.5%)
    Carotenids
    Flavonoids
    Volatile oil
    Steroidal saponins (capsicidins in seeds only)

    Key Actions:
    Stimulant
    Tonic
    Carminative
    Relieves muscle spasms
    Antispeptic sweating
    Increases sweating
    Increases blood flow to the skin
    Analgestic

16. *Carduus marianus* syn. *Silybum marianum* (Compositae)
    MILK THISTLE, MARY THISTLE
    A spiny biennial, growing to 1.5 m, with white-veined leaves and purple flowerheads.

    Key Constituents:
    Flavonlignans (1-4%) (silymarin)
    Bitter principles
    Polyacetylenes

    Key Actions:
    Protects the liver
    Stimlates secretion of bile
    Increases breast-milk production
    Antidepressant

17. *Cassia senna* syn. *Senna alexandrina* (Leguminosae)
    SENNA (ALEXANDRIAN SENNA)
    A small perennial shrub growing to 1 m, with straight

woody stem and yellow flowers.

Key Constituents:
Anthraquinine glycosides (sennosides)
Naphthalane glycosides
Mucilage
Flavonoids
Volatile oil

Key Actions:
Stimulant
Laxative
Cathartic

18. *Caulophyllum thalictroids* (Berberidaceae)
BLUE COHOSH, SQUAW ROOT, PAPOOSE ROOT
A perennial growing to 1 m, with large 3-lobed leaves, purple-blue flowers and deep blue berries.

Key Constituents:
Alkaloids (caulophylline, laburnine, magnoflorine)
Steroidal saponins (caulosapogenin)
Resin

Key Actions:
Antispasmodic
Diuretic
Promotes menstrual flow
Uterine tonic
Antirheumatic
Increasea sweating
Anti-inflammatory

19. *Centella asiatica* syn. *Hydrocotyle asiatica* (Umbelliferae)
GOTU KOLA (HINDI) INDIAN PENNYWORT
A perennial, herbaceous creeper, growing to 50 cm, with fan-shaped leaves.

Key constituents:
Riterpenoid saponins (asiaticocide, brahmoside thankuniside)
Alkaloids (hydrocotyline)

Bitter principies (Vellarin)

Key Actions:
Tonic
Antirheumatic
Mild diuretic
Sedative
Peripheral vasodilator

20. *Chamalirium luteum* syn. *Helonias dioica* (Liliaceae)
    HELONIAS, FALSE UNICORN ROOT, BLAZING STAR
    A herbaceous saponins (up to 9%)
    Glycosides (chamaelirin, helonin)

    Key Actions:
    Uterine & ovarion tonic
    Promotes menstrual flow
    Diuretic

21. *Chamomilla recutila* syn. *Matricaria recutita* (Compositae)
    GERMAN CHAMOMILE
    A sweetly aromatic annual growing to 60 cm, with finely cut
    leaves and white alowerheads.

    Key Constituents:
    Volatile oil (proazlenes, farnesine, alpha-bisabolol, spiroether)
    Flavonoids (anthemidin, luteolin, rutin)
    Bitter glycosides (anthemic acid)
    Coumarins
    Tannins

    Key Actions:
    Anti-inflammatory
    Antispasmodic
    Relaxant
    Carminative
    Mild bitter
    Anti-allergenic

22. *Chrysanthemum morifolium* (Compositae)
JU HUA (CHINESE), FLORISTS' CHRYSANTHEMUM
A perennial growing to about 1.5 m, with flowerheads composed of yellow ray floreste.

Key constituents:
Alkaloids including stachydrine
Volatile oil
Sesquiterpene lactones
Flavonoids, including apigenin
Betanine & choline
Vitamim 22

Key Actions:
Increase sweating
Antiseptic
Lowers blood pressure
Cooling
Reduces fever

23. *Cimicifuga racemosa* (Ranunculaceae).
BLACK COHOSH, SQUAW ROOT
A herbaceous perennial growing to about 2.5m, with creamy-white flower spikes.

Key constituents:
Triterpene glycosides (actein, cimicifugoside)
Isoflavones (formononetin)
Isoferulic acid
Salicylic acid

Key Actions:
Promotes menstrual flow
Antirheumatic
Expectorant
Sedative

24. *Cinchona spp.* (Rubiaceae)
CINCHONA, PERUVIAN BARK
An evergreen tree reaching 25 m, with reddish bark and leaves that grow to 50 cm.

Key Constituents:
Alkaloids (up to 15%), manily quinoline alkaloids (quinine,quinidine) and indole alkaloids (cinchonamine)
Bitter triterpenic glycosides (quinovin)
Tannins
Quinic acid

Key Actions:
Bitter
Reduces fever
Antimalarial
Tonic
Stimulates the appetile
Antispasmodic
Astringent
Antibacterial

25. *Cinnamomum verum* syn. *C. zeylanicum* (Lauraceae)
CINNAMON, DALCINI (HINDI)
An evergreen tree growing to 8-18 m, with soft, reddish brown bark and yellow flowers.

Key constituents:
Volatile oil up to 4% (Clinnamaldehyde 65-75%, eugenol 4-10%)
Tannins (condensed)
Coumarins
Mucilage

Key Actions:
Warning stumulant
Carminative
Antispasmodic
Antiseptic
Antiviral

26. *Citrus lemon* (Rutaceae)
LEMON
A small, evergreen tree growing to about 7 m, with light green, toothed leaves.

Key Constituents:
Volatile oil (about 2.5% fo the peel), limonene (up to 70%), alpha-terpinene, alpha-pinene, bete-pinene, citral. coumrins
Bioflavonoids
Vitamin A, B_1, B_2, B_3 and C (40-50mg per 100 g of fruit)
Mucilage

Key Actions:
Antiseptic
Antrihematic
Antibacterial
Antioxidant
Reduces Fever

27. *Codonopsis pilosula* (Campanulaceae)
    CODO NOPSIS, DANG SHEN (CHINESE)
    Codonopsis;
    A twinig perennial growing to 1.5 m with oval leaves and pendulous green and purple flowers.

Key constituents:
Triterpenoid saponins
Sterins
Alkenyl & alkenyl glycosides
Polysaccharides
Tangshenoiside I

Key Actions:
Adaptognic
Stimlant
Tonic

28. *Coleus forskohlil* syn. *Plectranthus barbatus* (Labiatae)
    COLEUS
    An aromatic perennial, with tuber-like roots and an erect stem, reaching 60 cm.

Key constituents:
Volatile oil
Diterpeners (forskolin)

Key Actions:
Lowers blood pressure
Antispasmodic
Dilates the bronchioles (small airways of the lungs)
Dilates the blood vessels
Heart tonic

29. *Commiphora molomol* syn. *C. myrrha* (Burseraceae)
    MYRRH
    A spiny, deciduous tree growing to 5 m, with yellow red flowers and pointed fruit.

Key Constituents:
Gum (30-60%), acidic polysaccharides
Resin (25-40%)
Volatile oil (308%), including heerabolene, eugenol and many furanosesquiterpenes.

Key Actions:
Stimulant
Antiseptic
Anti-inflammatory
Astringent
Expectorant
Antispasmodic
Carminative

30. *Corydalis yanhusuo* (Papaveraceae)
    CORYDALIS, YAN HU SUO (CHINESE)
    A small herbaceous plants growing to 30 cm with narrow leaves and pink flowers.

Key Constituents:
Alkaloids (including corydalisL, corydaline, Tetrahydro-palmatine (THP), protopine).
Protoberine-type alkaloid (leonticine)

Key Actions:
Analgesik
Antispasmodic
Sedative

31. *Crataegus oxyacantha & C. monogyna* (posaceae)
    HAWTHORM
    A deciduous, thorny tree with small leaves, white flowers and
    red berries, growing to 8 m.

    Key Constituents:
    Bioflavonoids (rutin, quercitin)
    Triterpenoids
    Cyanogenic glycosides
    Amines (trimenthylamine in flowers only)
    Polyphenols
    Coumarins
    Tannins

    Key Actions:
    Cardiotionic
    Dilates blood vessels
    Relaxant
    Antioxidant

32. *Crataeva nurvula* (Capparaceae)
    VARUNA, BARUN (HINDI), THREE-LEAFED CAPER
    A deciduous tree growing to 15 m, with pale yellow flowers.

    Key Constituents:
    Saponins
    Flavonoids
    Plant sterols
    Glucosilinates

    Key Actions:
    Diuretic
    Inhibits the formation of stones

33. *Curcuma longa syn. c. domestica* (Zingiberaceae)
    TURMERIC, HALDI (HINDI), JIANG HUANG (CHINESE)
    A perennial reaching 90 cm, with a short stem, lanceshaped
    leaves and knobbly rhizome.

    Key Constituents:
    Volatile oil (3-5%), including zingiberin and turmerone

Curcumin
Bitter principles
Resin

Key Actions:
Stimulates secretion of bile
Anti-inflammatory
Eases stomach pain
Antioxidant
Antibacterial

34. *Dioscorea villosa* (Dioscoreaceae)
WILD YAM
A deciduous perennial vine, climbing to 6 m, with heartshaped leaves and tiny green flowers.

Key Constituents:
Steroidal saponins (mainly dioscin)
Phytosterols
Alkaloids
Tannins
Starch

Key Actions:
Antispasmodic
Anti-inflammatory
Antirheumatic
Increases sweating
Diuretic

35. *Echinacea anqustifolia & E. purpurea* (Compositae)
ECHINACEA, PURPLE CONEFLOWER
Echinacea:
A perennial growing to 50 cm, with daisy-like purple flowers, and leaves covered in coarse hair.

Key Constituents:
Alkamaides (mostly isobutylamides with olefinic and acety-lenic bonds)
Caffeic acid esters (mainly echinacoside and cynarin)
Polysaccharides

Volatile oil (humulene)
Echinolone
Betanine

Key Actions:
Immune stimulant
Anti-inflammatory
Antibiotic
Detoxifying
Increases sweating
Heals
Anti-allergenic

36. *Elettaria cardamomum* (Zingiberaceae)
CARDAMOM, ELACHI (HINDI)
A perennial growing to 5 m, with mauve-marked, white flowers and very long lance-shaped leaves.

Key Constituents:
Volatile oil (borneol, camphor, pinene, humulene, caryophyllene, carvone, eucalyptole, terpinene, sabinene).

Key Actions:
Eases stomach pain
Carminative
Aromatic
Warming digestive stimulant
Antispasmodic

37. *Eleutherococcus senticosus* (Araliaceae)
SIBERIAN GINSENG
A deciduosu, hardy shurb, growing to 3 m. It has 3-7 toothed leaflets on each stem.

Key Constituents:
Eleutherosides, 0.6-0.9%
Phenylpropanoids
Lignans
Sugars
Polysaccharides
Triterpenoid saponins

Glycans

Key Actions:
Adaptogenic
Tonic
Stimulant
Protects the immune system

38. *Ephedra sinica* (Ephedraceae)
    EPHEDRA, MA HUANG (CHINESE), DESERT TEA
    An evergreen shrub growing to 60 cm, with long narrow
    sprawing stems and tiny leaves.

    Key Constituents:
    Protoalkaloids (ephedrine, pseudoephedrine)
    Tannins
    Saponin
    Flavone
    Volatile oil

    Key Actions:
    Western herbal medicine:
    Increases sweating
    Dilates 'he bronchioles (small airways in the lungs)
    Diuretic
    Stimulant
    Raises blood pressure
    Chinese herbal medicine:
    Disperses cold
    Helps problems caused by "external cold"
    Aids movement of lung qi

39. *Eucalyptus globulus* (Myrtaceae)
    EUCALYPTUS, BLUE GUM
    An evergreen tree growing to 100 m, with a blue-grey trunk
    and green leaves.

    Key Constituents:
    Volatile oil (cineole; up to 80%)
    Flavonoids
    Tannins

Resin

Key Actions:
Antiseptic
Expectorant
Stimulates local blood flow

40. *Elugenia caryophyllata syn. Syzyium aromaticum* (Myrtaceae)
CLOVE
An evergreen, pyramid-shaped tree growing to 15 m. The tree
is strongly aromatic.

Key Constituents:
Volatile oil containing eugenol (up to 85%), acetyl eugenol,
methyl salicylate, pinene, vanillin
Gum
Tannins

Key Actions:
Antiseptic
Carminative
Stimulant
Analgesic
Prevents vomiting
Antispasmodic
Eliminates parasites

41. *Filipendula ulmaria* (Rosaceae)
MEADOWSWEET, QUEEN OF THE MEADOW
A perennial reaching 1.5 m, with toothed leaves and clusters
of creamy, scented flowers.

Key Constituents:
Flavonol glycosides (approximately 1%), mainly glycosides of
quercetin
Phenolic glycosides (salicylates)
Volatile oil (salicylaldehyde)
Polyphenols (tannins)

42. *Gentiana lutea* (Gentianaceae)
GENTIAN:
An erect perennial growing t 1.2 m, with starshaped yellow flowers and oval leaves.

Key Constituents:
Bitter principles (gentiopicroside, amarogentin)
Gentianose
Inulin
Pectin
Phenolic acids

Key Actions:
Bitter
Digestive stimulant
Eases stomach pain

43. *Ginkgo biloba* (Ginkgoaceae)
GINKGO, MAIDENHAIR TREE, BAI GUO (CHINESE)
A deciduous tree with one or several main trunks and spreading branches. It grows to 30 m.

Key Constituents:
Flavonoids
Ginkgolides
Bilobalides

Key Actions:
Circulatory stimulant & tonic
Anti-asthmatic
Antispasmodic
Anti-allergenic
Anti-inflammatory

44. *Glycyrrhiza glabra* (Leguminosae)
LIQUORICE
A woody-stemmed perennial growing to 2 m, with dark leaves and cream to mative flowers.

Key Constituents:
Triterene saponins (glycyrrhizin, up to 6%)
Flavonoids (isoflavones: liquiritin, isoliquiritin, formononetin)

Polysaccharides
Sterols
Coumarins
Asparagin

Key Actions:
Anti-inflammatory
Expectorant
Demulcent
Adrenal agent
Mild laxative

45. *Hamamelis virginiana* (Hamamelidaceae)
WITCH HAZEL
A small deciduous tree growing to 5 m (15 ft), with coarsely toothed, broadly oval leaves.

Key Constituents:
Tannins (8-10%)
Flavonoids
Bitter priciple
Volatile oil (leaves only)

Key Actions:
Astringent
Anti-inflammatory
Stops external and internal bleeding

46. **Harpagophytum procumben (Pedaliaceae)**
DEVIL'S CLAW
A trailing perennial, reaching 1.5 m in length, with fleshy lobed leaves and barbedm woody fruit.

Key Constituents:
Iriboid glycosides (harpago side)
Sugars (stachyose)
Phytosterols
Flavonoids
Harpagoquinone

Key Actions:
Anti-inflammatory

Analgesic
Digestive stimulant

47. *Humulus lupulus* (Cannabaceae)
HOPS
A tall, clibing perennial, growing to 7 m. Hop plants are either male or female.

Key Constituents:
Bitter principles (lupulin containing humulon, lupulon and valerianic acid)
Volatile oil (1%), humulene
Flavonoids
Polyphenolic tannins
Oestrogenic substances
Asparagin

Key Action:
Sedative
Soporific
Antispasmodic
Aromatic bitter

48. *Hydrastis canadensis* (Ranunculaceae)
GOLDENSEAL
A small herbaceous perennial, with a thick yellow root and an erect stem growing to 30cm.

Key Constituents:
Isoquinoline alkaloids (hydrastine, berberine, canadine)
Volatile oil
Resin

Key Actions:
Tonic
Mild laxative
Anti-inflammatory
Antibacterial
Bitter
Uterine stimulant Stops internal bleeding
Astringent

49. *Hypericum perforatium* (Guttiferae)
ST JOHN'S WORT, Y FENDIGEDIG (WELSH)
An erect perennial growing to 80 cm, with bright yellow
flowers in a flat-topped cluster.

Key Constituents:
Volatile oil (carophyllene)
Hypericin & pseudohypericin
Flavonoids

Key Actions:
Antidepressant
Antispasmodic
Stimulates bile flow
Astringent
Sedative
Relieves pain
Antiviral

50. *Inula helenium* (Compositae)
ELECAMPANE
A perennial growing to 3 m, with golden yellow, daisylike
flowers and large pointed leaves.

Key Constituents:
Inulin (up to 44%)
Volatile oil (up to 4%), containing alantol and sesquiterpene
lactones (including alantolactone)
Triterpene saponins (dammaranedienol)
Sterols
Polyacetylenes

Key Actions:
Expectorant
Soothes coughing
Increases sweating
Mildly bitter
Eliminates worms
Antiseptic

51. *Jateorhiza palmata* syn. *J. calumba* (Menispermaceae)
CALUMBA
A twining perennial growing to 15 m, with large palmlike leaves and green-white flowers.

Key Constituents:
Isoquinoline alkaloids (palmatine, columbamine, jatrorrhizine)
Bitter principles (furaniditerpenol, palmanin)
Volatile oil (up to 1% - mostly thymol)
Mucilage

Key Actions:
Bitter
Eases stomach pain
Tonic
Reduces fever
Expels worms

52. *Lavandula officinalis* syn. *angustifolia* (Labiatae)
LAVENDER
A perender shurb growing to 1 m, with spikes of violet-blue flowers extending above the foliage.

Key Constituents:
Volatile oil (up to 3%) containing over 40 constituents, including linalyl acetate (30-60%), cineole (10%), linalool, nerol, borneol
Flavonoids
Tannins
Coumarins

Key Actions:
Carminative
Relieves muscle spasms
Antidepresant
Antiseptic & antibacterial
Stimulates blood flow

53. *Lobelia inflata* (Campanulaceae)
LOBELIA, INDIAN TOBACCO
An annual growing to 50 cm, with lance-shaped leaves and pale blue, pink-tinged flowers.

Key Constituents:
Piperidine alkaloids (principally lobeline, but many others present)
Carboxyylic acids

Key Actions:
Respiratory stimulant
Antispasmodic
Expectorant
Induces vomiting
Increaces sweating

54. *Lycium Chinense* (Solanaceae)
LYCIUM, CHINESE WOLFBERY
A deciduous shurb growing to 4m, with bright green leaves and scarlet berries.

Key Constituents:
Berries only
Physalien
Carotene
Vitamins B_1, B_{12} and C
Root only
Cinnamic acid
Psyllic acid

Key Actions:
Berries
Tonic
Protect the liver
Root
Reduces fever
Lowers blood pressure

55. *Melaleuca alternifolia* (Myrtaceae)
TEA TREE
An evergreen reaching 7 m, with layers of papery bark, pointed leaves and white flower spikes.

Key Constituents:
Volatile oil (percentages are variable), terpinen-4-01 40%,

gammmaterpinene 24%, alpha-terpinene 10%, cineol 5%.

Key Actions:
Antiseptic
Antibacterial
Antifungal
Antiviral
Immune stimulant

56. *Melissa officinalis* (Labiatae)
LEMON BALM? BALM
A perennial growing to 1.5 m, with tiny white flowers and
deeply veined, toothed leaves.

Key Constituents:
Volatile oil up to 0.2% (citral, caryophyllene oxide, linalool
and citronellal)
Flavonoids
Triterpenes
Polyphenols
Tannins

Key Actions:
Relaxant
Antispasmodic
Increases sweating
Carminative
Antiviral
Nerve tonic

57. *Mentha piperita* (Labiatae)
PEPPERMINI
A strongly aromatic, square-stemmaed annual, growing to 80
cm with serrated leaves.

Key Constituents:
Volatile oil (up to 1.5%), including menthol (35-55%), menthone
(10-40%) Flavonoids (luteolin, menthoside)
Phoenolic acids
Triterpenes

Key Actions:
Carminative
Relieves muscle spasms
Increases sweating
Stimulates secretion of bile
Antiseptic

58. *Myristica fragrans* (Myristicaceae)
NUTMEG & MACE ROU DOU KOU (CHINESE)
Nutmeg tree growing to 12 m, with aromatic leaves and clusters of small yellow flowers.

Key Constituents:
Numeg;
Volatile oil (up to 15%), including alpha-pinene, beta-pinene, alpha-terpine, beta-terpinene, myristicin, elincin, safrole.
Fixed oil (nutmeg better:), myristine, butyrin
Mace;
Volatile oil (similar to nutmeg but with a higher concentration of myristicin).

Key Actions:
Nutmeg   Mace
Carminative
Stimulant
Relives muscle spasms
Carminative
Prevents vomiting
Stimulant

59. *Ocimum sanctum* (Labiatae)
HOLY BASIL, TULSI (HINDI)
An aromatic annual growing to about 70 cm, with small, purple-red or white flowers.

Key Constituents:
Volatile oil (1%) including eugenol (70-80%), methyl-chavicol, methyl eugenol, caryophyllene.
Flavonoids (apigenin, uteolin)
Triterpene (ursolic acid)

Key Actions:
Lowers blood sugar levels
Antispaamodic
Analgesic
Lowers blood pressure
Redues fever
Adaptogenic
Anti-inflammatory

60. *Paeonia lactiflora* syn. *p. albiflore* (Paeoniaceae)
WHITE PEONY, BAI SHAO YAO (CHINESE)
An epright perennial, growing to 2 m, with large white flowers and divided, dark green laeves,

Key Constituents:
Monoterpenoid glycosides (paeoniflorin, albiflorin)
Benzolic acid
Pentagalloyl glucose

Key Actions:
Antispasmodic
Tonic
Astringent
Antgesic

61. *Panax ginseng* (Araliaceae)
GINSENG, REN SHEN (CHINESE)
A perennial growing to 1m, with oval, toothed leaves and a cluster of small green-yellow flowers.

Key Constituents:
Triterpenoid saponins (0.7-3%), ginsenosides-at least 25 have been identified
Acetylenic compounds
Panaxans
Seequiterpenes

Key Actions:
Adaptogenic
Tonic

62. **Passiflora incarnata** (Passifloraceae)
    PASSION FLOWER, PASSIFLORA, MAYPOP
    A climbing vine growing to 9 m, with 3-lobed leaves, ornate
    flowers and egg-shaped fruit.

    Key Constituents:
    Flavonoids (apigenin)
    Meltrol
    Cyanogenic glycosides (gynocardin)
    Indole alkaloids (harman)

    Key Actions:
    Sedative
    Antispasmodic
    Tranquillizing.

63. **Persea americana** (Lauracaea)
    AVOCADO
    An evergreen tree, growing to 20 m, with dark green, leathery
    leaves and white flowers.

    Key Constituents:
    Leaves & bark
    Volatile oil (methylchvicol, alpha-pinene)
    Flavonoids
    Tannins
    Fruit pulp
    Unsaturated fats
    Protein (about 25%)
    Sesquiterpenes
    Vitamins A, B_1, and B_2

    Key Action:
    Leaves & bark
    Astringent
    Carminative
    Relieve coughs
    Promote menstrual flow

64. ***Piper methysticum*** (Piperaceae)
KAVA KAVA
An evergreen shrub climbing to 3 m, with fleshy stems and heart-shaped leaves.

Key Constituents:
Resin containing kava lactones, including kawain
Piperidine alkaloid (pipermethysticine)

Key Actions:
Stimulant
Tonic
Reduces anxiety
Urinary antiseptic
Analgesic Induces sleep

65. ***Plantago spp.*** (Plantaginaceae)
PSYLLIUM, ISPAGHULA (HINDI), FLEA SEED
An annual, growing to 40 cm high, with narrow leaves and clusters of minure white-brown flowers.

Key Constituents:
Mucilage (arabinoxylan)
Fixed oil (2.5%) - mainly linoleic, oleic and palmitic fatty acids
Starch

Key Actions:
Demulcent
Bulk laxative
Antidiarrhoeal

66. ***Polygonum multiflorium*** (Polygonaceae)
HE SHOU WU (CHINESE)? FLOWERY KNOTWEED
A perennial climber, growing to 10 m, with red stems, light green leaves and white or pink flowers.

Key Constituents:
Chrysophanic acid
Anthraquinones (emodin, rhein)
Lecithin

Key Actions:
Mildly sedative
Nourishes the blood
Tonic

67. *Prunella vulgaris* (Labiatae)
SELF-HEAL, XU KU CAO (CHINESE)
A creeping perennial, growing to 50 cm, with pointed oval leaves and violet-blue or pink flowers.

Key Constituents:
Pentacyclic triterpenes (based on ursolic, betulinic and oleanolic acids)
Tannins
Caffeic acid
Vitamins B_1, C, K

Key Actions:
Heals wounds
Astringent
Stops internal bleeding
Gently lowers blood pressure

68. *Rehmannia glutinosa* (Scrophulariaceae)
REHMANNIA, DI HUANG (CHINESE)
A perennail, reaching 30-60 cm, with large, sticky leaves and purple flowers.

Key Constituents:
Phytosterols (beta-sitosterol, stigmasterol)
Sugars (mannitol)
Rehmannin

Key Actions:
Tonic
Kidney tonic
Lowers blood pressure
Protects the liver

69. **Rheum palmatium** (Polygonaceae)
   CHINESE RHUBARB, DA HUANG (CHINESE)
   A thick-rhizomed perennial growing to 3 m, with large palm-shaped leaves and small flowers.

   Key Constituents:
   Anthraqioones (about 3-5%), rhein, aleo-emodin, emodin
   Lavonoids (catechin)
   Phenolic acids
   Tannins (5-10%)
   Calcium oxalate

   Key Actions:
   Laxative
   Constipating
   Astringent
   Eases stomach pain
   Antibacterial.

70. **Rosmarinus officinalls** (Labiatae)
   ROSEMARY
   A storngly aromatic evergreen shurb growing to 2 m, with narrow, dark green, pine-like leaves.

   Key Constituents:
   Volatile oil (1-2%) containing borneol, camphene camphor, cineole
   Flavonoids (apigenin, diosmin)
   Tannins
   Rosmarinic acid
   Diterpenes (picrosalvin)
   Rosmaricine

   Key Actions:
   Tonic
   Stimulant
   Astringent
   Nervine
   Anti-inflammatory
   Carminative

71. *Rumex crispus* (Polygonaceae)
    YELLOW DOCK, CURLED DOCK
    A perennial growing from 30 cm to 1.5 m, with lance-shaped
    leaves up to 25 cm (10 im) long.

    Key Constituents:
    Anthraquinones (up to 4%), nepodin, emodin, chrysaphanol
    Tannins
    Oxalates
    Volatile oil

    Key Actions:
    Mild laxative
    Stimulates bile flow
    Cleansing

72. *Sabal Serrulata syn. Serenoa serrulata* (Palmaceae)
    SAW PALMETTO
    A small palm growing to 6 m, with fans of yellow-green leaves
    and ivory flowers.

    Key Constituents:
    Volatile Oil (1-2%)
    Fixed oil
    Steroidal saponin
    Polysaccharides
    Tannins

    Key Actions:
    Tonic
    Diuretic
    Sedative
    Anabolic
    Oestrogenic

73. *Salix alba* (Salicaceae)
    WHITE WILLOW
    A deciduous tree growing to 25 m (80 ft), with green tapering
    leaves, and catkins in spring.

Key Constituents:
Phenolic glycosides (up to 11%) - salicylic acid
Flavonoids
Tannins (up to 20%)

Key Actions:
Anti-inflammatory
Analgesic
Reduces fever
Antirheumatic
Astringent

74. *Salvia multiorrhiza* (Labiatae)
DAN SHEN, RED SAGE
A hardly perennial growing to 80 cm, with toothed oval leaves and clusters of purple flowers.

Key Constituents:
Tanshinones
Tanshinol
Salviol
Vitamin E
Volatile Oil

Key Actions:
Circulatory tonic
Dilates the blood vessels
Sedative
Antibacterial

75. *Salvia officinalis* (Labiatae)
SAGE
An evergreen growing to 80 cm (32 m), with square stems and hairy grey-green or purple leaves

Key constituents:
Volatile Oil (thujone-about 50%)
Diterpene bitters
Flavonoids
Phenolic acids
Tannins

Key Actions:
Astringent
Antiseptic
Aromatic
Carminative
Oestrogenic
Reduces sweating
Tonic

76. ***Sambucus nigra*** (Caprifoliaceae)
ELDER
A deciduous tree growing to 10 m, with oval leaves, cream flowers and blue-black berries.

Key Constituents:
Flowers:
Flavonoids (up to %) - rutin
Phenolic acids
Triterpenes
Sterols
Volatile oil (up to 0.2%)
Mucilage
Tannins
Leaves
Cyanogenic glycosides
Berries
Flavonoids
Anthocyanins
Vitamins A and C

Key Actions:
Increases sweating
Diuretic
Anti-inflammatory

77. ***Schisandra chinensis*** (Schisandraceae)
SCHISANDRA, WU WEI ZI (CHINESE)
An aromatic woody vine reaching up to 8 m, with pink flowers and spikes of red berries.

Key Constituents:
Lignans (schizandrin, deoxyschizandrin, gomisin)
Phytosterols (beta-sitosterol, stigmalterol)
Volatile oil
Vitamins C and E
Key Actions
Tonic
Adaptogenic
Protects liver

78. *Scutellaria baicalensis syn. S. Macrantha* (Labiatae)
BAICAL SKULLCAP, HUANG QUIN
A perennial growing to 30-120 cm hight, with lance-shaped leaves and purplish-blue flowers.

Key Constituents:
Flavonoids (about 12%) - baicalin, wogoniside
Sterols
Benzoic acid

Key Actions:
Sedative
Anti-allergenic
Antibiotic
Anti-inflammatory

79. *Scutellaria lateriflora* (Labiatae)
SKULLCAP, VIRGINIAN SKULLCAP, MAD DOG
A perennial growing to 60 cm, with an erect, many-branched stem and pink to blue flowers.

Key Constituents:
Flavonoids (scutellarin)
Bitter iridoids (catalpol)
Volatile oil
Tannins

Key Actions:
Sadevtive
Nervine tonic
Antispasmodic
Mild bitter

80. *Swetia Chirata syn. Ophelia Chirata* (Gentianaceae)
    CHIRETTA;
    An annual growing to about 1 m. Hight with smooth leaves
    and purple-tinged, pale green flowers.

    Key Constituents:
    Xanthones
    Iridoids (including amarogentin)
    Alkaloids
    Flavones

    Key Actions:
    Biteer
    Tonic
    Stimulates the appetic
    Eases stomach pain
    Reducec fever
    Antimalarial

81. *Symphatum officinale* (Boraginaceae)
    COMFERY, KNITBONE
    A perennial growing to 1 m, with thick leaves and bell-like
    white to pink or mauve flowers

    Key Constituents:
    Allanotin (up to 4.7%)
    Muscilage (about 29%)
    Triterpenoids
    Phenolic acids (rosmarinic acid)
    Asparagine
    Pyrrolizidine alkaloids (0.02-0.07%) Tannins

    Key Actions:
    Demulent
    Astingent
    Anti-inflammatory
    Heals wound and bones

82. *Syzygium cumini* (Myrtacaea)
    JAMBUL
    An evergreen tree growing to 10 m, with lance-shaped leaves

and green-yellow flowers.

Key Constituents:
Phenols (methylxanthoxylin)
Tannins
Alkaloid (jumbosine)
Triterpenoids
Volatile oil

Key Actions:
Lowers blood sugar levels
Astringent
Carminative
Diuretic

83. *Tabebuia spp.* (Bignoniaceae)
LAPACHO (SPANISH), PAU D'ARCO (PORTUGUESE)
An evergreen tree (deciduous in cold climates) reaching 30 cm
(100 ft), with pink flowers.

Key Constituents:
Quinoners (lapachol)
Bioflavonoids
Lapachenole
Carnosal
Indoles
Coenzyme Q
Alkaloids (tecommine)
Steroidal Saponins

Key Actions:
Antibiotic
Antifungal
Immune-stimulant
Anti-inflammatory
Cleansing
Tonic
Anti-tumour

84. ***Tanacetum parthenium*** (Compositae)
FEVERFEW
A herbicious perennial growing to 60 cm, with numerous daisy-like flowerheads.

Key Constituents:
Volatile oil (alpha-pinene)
Sesquiterpene lactones (parthenolide)
Sesquiterpenes (camphor)

Key Actions:
Analgesic
Reduces fever
Antriheumatic
Promotes menstrual flow
Bitter

85. ***Taraxacum officinale*** (Compositae)
DANDELION
A perennial growing to 50 cm, with ragged basal leaves, hollow stalks and golden flowers.

Key Constituents:
Sesquiterpene lactiones
Triterpenes
Vitamins A, B, C, and D
Leaf only
Coumarins
Carotenoids
Minerals (especially potassium)
Root only
Taraxacoside
Phenolic acids
Mineral (potassium, calcium)

Key Actions:
Diuretic
Detoxifying
Bitter

86. *Terminalia arjuna* (Combertaceae)
ARJUNA
An evergreen tree reaching 30 m, with pale yellow flowers and cone-shaped leaves.

Key Constituents:
Tannins
Triterpenoid saponins
Flavonoids
Sterols

Key Actions:
Cardiac tonic
Lower blood pressure
Reduces cholesterol levels

87. *Thymus vulgaris* (Labittae)
THYME, GARDEN THYME
An aromatic shurb growing to 40 cm, with woody stams, small leaves and pink flowers.

Key Constituents:
Volatile oil with varible content (thymol, methylchavicol, cineole, borneol)
Flavonoids (spinanin, luteleoin)
Tannins

Key Actions:
Antiseptic
Tonic
Relieves muscle pains
Expectorant
Expels worms

88. *Turnera diffusa syn. T. diffusa var. aphrodisiaca* (Turneraceae)
DAMIANA
An aromatic shurb growing to 2 m, with smooth, pale green leaves and small, single yellow flowers.

Key Constituents:
Arbutin (up to 7%)
Volatile oil (about 0.5%), delacadinene (100%), thymol (4%)

Cyanogenic glycoside (tetraphyllin)
Resin
Gums

Key Actions:
Tonic
Stimulant
Mild laxative & diuretic
Antidepresant
Testosterogenic
Reputed aphrodisiac

91. *Ulmus rubra* (Ulmaceae)
SLIPPERY ELM
A large tree growing to 18 m with a brown trunk and rough
grey-white bark on the branches.

Key Constituents:
Mucilage
Starch
Tannins

Key Actions:
Demulcent
Emollient
Nutritive
Laxative

92. *Urtica dioica* (Urticaceae)
NETTLE
A perennial growing to 1.5 m, with lance-sharped leaves and
green flowers with yellow stamens.

Key Constituents:
Aerial parts
Flavonoids (quercitin)
Amines (histamine, choline, acetylcholine, serotonin)
Glucoquinone
Minerals (calcium, potassium, silicic acid, iron)
Root

Phenols

Key Actions:
Diuretic
Tonic
Astringent
Prevents haemorhaging
Anti-allergenic
Increase breast-milk (production leaf)
Reduces prostate enlargement (root)

93. *Valeriana officinalis* (Valerianaceae)
VALERIAN
Erect perenneal growing to 1.2 m, with pinnate divided leaves
and pink flowers.

Key Constituents:
Volatile oil (up to 1.4%), including bornyl acetate, beta-caryphyllene
Indoids (valepotriates) - valtrate, isovaltrate
Alkaloids

Key Actions:
Sedative
Relaxant
Relieves muscle spasms
Relieves anxiety
Lowers blood pressure

94. *Verbena officianlis* (Verbenaceae)
VERVAIN, MA BIAN CAO (CHINESE)
A slender perennial growing to 1 m (3 ft), with stiff, then stems
and spikes of small like flowers.

Key Constituents:
Bitter iridoids (verberin, verbenalin)
Volatile oil
Alkaloids
Mucilage
Tennins

Key Actions:
Nervine
Tonic
Mild sedative
Stimulates bile secretion
Mild bitter

EXAMPLES IN PHARMACOGNOSY

1. COLCHICUM

Colchicum luteum — Yields the commercial colchicum corm. The liliaceous plant is an annual herb found in North Western Himalayas, in outskirts of forests or open grassy places. Leaves very narrow but broader towards the tip. Flowers large. *Colchicum autumnale* is a variety that grows throughout Europe.

Cultivation — The seeds are sown in September on thin soil. Germination is observed at the onset of winter or in the early spring. When one year old, the underground rhizome parts take their shape and they are transplanted in the field. The distance between the plants should be 60 cm apart. The plant shows flower in August or September after three years. The leaves show a rosette of large lanceolate type 15-25 cm long. The leaves die down in July and in the September the crocus like purple flowers appear.

After 4-5 years the rhizomes take corm like structure which is covered by fibrous roots and membranous scales.

Collection — The corms are lifted from the ground. The roots and membranous portions should be cleared. Then the corm may be used fresh or may be dried.

Description of the corm

Corms are brownish in colour, almost conical in shape with one side flat, the other roundish. The outer surface of the corm is marked by indefinite and irregular longitudinal striactions. Corms are 30-45 mm long, 15-25 mm wide and 7-15 mm thick.

Internal structure

The outermost structure (i.e. epidermis) is consisting of tubular polygonal cells about 58-80µ wide, 90-140µ long and 16-20µ high. In European variety, the epidermal cells contain occasional stomata. Next layers are consisting of thin layered parenchyma cells filled with starch grains which are gelatinised. The vascular bundles are slender, collateral and scattered, xylem vessels are spiral. The starch grains are simple, rounded or compound with two or three components. The hilum is central and is either a point or a two to three radiate split. The alkaloid colchicine is present in the epidermis and in a sheath, surrounding each vascular bundle.

Chemical Constituents

The fresh corms of the plant collected before its flowering constitute the drug *Colchicum corm* and in the ripe dried ·ds, the drug *Colchicum* seed. The alkaloid colchicine is toxic and dried corm contains upto 0.6 percent colchicine. Indian variety is poorer in contents but contains abudance of starch.

Uses—The active principle colchicine is useful in pains and inflammations of goat. The use of the drug can, however, cause severe irritation in the intestine.

Other uses—Colchicine has been largely used in scientific research in animals and plants. The effect of colchicine on cancerous tissue has been tested and the drug arrests division of cells of the cancerous tissue and also makes them more susceptible to x-ray treatments. Colchicine induces polyploidy in seedlings treated with a weak solution. It arrests the spindle formation at metaphase of mitosis.

2. IPECAC

I. Ipecacuanha

Cephaelis ipecacuanha A Rubiaceous trailing herbaceous plant is a native of Brazil in South America and is cultivated in India (in Assam, Bengal and on an Experimental scale in South India). The dried adventitious roots of the plant commercially known as ipecacuanha root. *Cephalis acuminata* is known as Panama ipecac.

Cultivation—The Ipecac plantation in West Bengal has been developed as the largest in the world. The soil best suited for cultivation of ipecac is a sandy loam, rich in humous. Further, the yield becomes greater, if there is a good percentage of ashes, magnesium or lime present in the soil. The soil should be well-drained and have annual rainfall of about 2.5 m and the temperature should be ranging between 10-20°C. The plants are grown by means of root cuttings and planted a metre apart. Propagation is done by means of seeds, but in such cases, the growth of the plants is rather slow.

Collection—The plants are low, straggling shrubs with slender rhizomes bearing annulated roots. As they grow in clumps, a group is lifted from the soil by inserting a pointed stick beneath them. The adhering soil is shaken off and the roots are dried in the sun (not exceeding 65°C). The drug is during dry season.

Description of Ipecacuanha

The surface of the root is dark brown. It is slender 4-7mm long, 3-5 mm thick and is marked by transverse constriction that gives the appearance of annulations.

The stem is uniformly cylindrical structure associated with root.

Internal Structure of Ipecacuanha (Root)

The transverse cut surface shows a central core of yellowish white wood surrounded by cambium line and thin brown cork externally. The primary xylem is triarch surrounded by secondary xylem traversed by medullary rays. The medullary rays may be one or two. The cambium is normal bearing xylem inside and phloem outside. The phloem occurs in small groups embedded in parenchymatous phelloderm which occupies large arears. Beyond this is a narrow layer of cork. the xylem is consisting of bordered pitted tracheids, vessels, and xylem parenchyma. The last structure is also consisting of simple pits and contains starch grains as reserve food. The starch grains are compound and each grain measures 4-10μ in diameter.

The phelloderm carries scattered idioblast cells each of which contains a bundle of a circular raphides of calcium oxalate crystals being about 30-80μ long. The corky layer is consisting of phellogen and bark. The bark is horny in appearance with starch and the cork is thin and brown. The central portion is occupied by pith. Large vessels, phloem fibres and sclerieds are absent in root. The xylem parenchyma with simple pits substitutes the fibres. The annulations show the presence of cambium.

The internal structure of stem present in the drug shows same internal structure like root. The pith is parenchymatous and pericycle is sclerenchymatous. The external structure to the cortex is the cork. The interstelar region is consisting of phloem cambium and xylem

Chemical Constituents

Ipecacuanha root contains 3 principal alkaloids in the bark and makes up about 90% of the drug.

(a) *Emetine*—A white odorless, crystalline powder is present in about 66-72% of the total content. Emetine hydrochloride is a hydrated hydrochloride of emetine. It is soluble in water and alcohol.

(b) Cephaline — A phenolic alkaloid and is present about 26% of the total content.

(c) Psychrotine — A phenolic alkaloid.

There are two more alkaloids-emetamine and methyl-psychotrine.

There are other constituents like glycosides (ipecacuanbin), starch (30-40%), calcium oxalate, acid saponin and ipecacuanhic acid.

The stem portion contains the same alkaloids as the root but usually in smaller portion.

Uses—It is used largely in the form of syrup as an expectorant and emetic. The drug mixed with opium acts as diaphoretic. The emetic properties act as antidote in poison. It is also used as a remedy for amoebic dysentry (emetine hydrochloride).

Varieties—Indian ipecacuanha-contains 50% alkaloid emetine. The colour of the powder is bright and shape is large.

Brazilian ipecacuanha or (Rio)—The alkaloid contents are lesser and out of total alkaloid about 1/3rd is cephaeline and 2/3rd emetine.

Cartagena ipecacuanha (Colombo)—The total alkaloid content reaches 2.2%. The variety is referred as Cephaelis acuminata. Annulations are not present.

Panama ipecacuanha—The alkaloid content is 2.2%.

Nicaragua ipecacuanha—The total alkaloid content is 2.5% out of which emetine is 20-25%.

Minas ipecacuanha—The total alkaloid content is 2.2% but the proportion of emetine is about 60%. It is a commercial variety of Rhio ipecacuanha.

Test for emetine—To Freshly powdered root 0.5gm is taken for the test. Then a solution is made with the powder mixed with 20ml concentrated HCl and 5ml of water. The mixture is filtered and 2ml is taken. Then 0.01gm of potassium chlorate is added. The mixture takes yellow colour, changes to red after an hour.

This test may be observed in cut surface of root. The transverse cut surface shows a central core of yellowish white dense wood. If the sections are exposed in air or in the sun, the colour changes to red.

Substitutes—There are six substitutes of Ipecacuanha, namely *Cryptocoryne spiralis* (Araceae) known as East Indian root (stele parenchymatous, and white starchy cortex);

Richardsonia scabra (Rubiaceae) known as undulated ipecacuanha (porus wood, starchy bark); *Manettia ignita* (Rubiaceae) known as lesser straited ipecacuanha (stouter aerial stem, starchy violet bark); *Psychotria emetica* (Rubiaceae) known as greater straiated ipecacuanha (dark violet bark, starch absent) *Hybanthus ipecacuanha* (Violacee) known as white ipecacuanha (darker bark, yellowish wood) and *Asclepias curasserica* (Asclepiadaceae) known as Trinidad ipecacuanha (unplesant bitter taste.)

Important alkaloid containing barks

(BARK)

Source	Chemical Constituents	Uses	Substitutes
Cinnamon bark (*Cinnanamum zeylanicum*) Fam-Lauraceae cultivated in Srilanka	Volatile oil, tannin and mucilage	Carminative, aromatic and antiseptic	C. *loureiril*, C. *oliveri*
Slippery elm bark (*Ulmus fleva-Ulmaceae*, a small tree of United States	Mucilage which does not dissolve in water	External application form of a poultice	
Alder Buchthorn bark (*Fraggula alnus* Rhamnaceae)	Glycoside, franjulin	Laxative	*Rhamnus carmiolica Alrus glutinosa Betulaceae*
Quillaia bark (*Quilaya saponaria* Rosaceae)	Toxic glycoside (quillajic acid and quillaia sepotoxin)	Stimulant and expectorant	
Cinchona (*Cinchona sp.*)		Fibres short-radial rows, 25.90m wide, microcrystals in idioblasts, crystals 2-6µ long, stone cells absent, starch grains small, bitter	

(Contd.)

Name	Characters
Cassia (*Cinnamomum cassia*)	Fibres in short tangential rows, 30µ width, calcium oxalate needle shaped, scattered stone cells numerous, starch grains abundant aromatic, oil and mucilage present.
Alstonia (*Alstonia scholaris*)	Fibres isolated, prismatic crystals of calcium oxalate Epidermal trichomes absent cork thin walled, starch in medullary rays, latex tube present.

Some important members with histological characters

(LEAF)

Name	Characters
Foxglove (*Digitalis purpurea*)	Stomata on the upper surface few, lower numerous, calcium oxalate present, trichome 3-5 cells long, glandular, mesophylls not differentiated, water pores present.
Xanthium (*Xanthium strumarium*)	Stomata *Ranunculus* type, trichomes few, conical, calcium oxalate absent, mesophyll differentiated effervescence with acid.
Belladona (*Atropa belladonna*)	Stomata on the upper surface few, lower surface many, Cruciferous type, trichome uniseriate, calcium crystals present, mesophylls differentiated.
Phytolacca (*Phytolacea decandra*)	Stomata on the lower surface upper surface nil, trichome absent, mesophyll differentiated, calcium oxalate in idioblasts.
Coca (*Erythroxylum coca*)	Stomata on the lower surface, upper surface nil, calcium oxalate in crystals, trichomes absent, mesophyll differentiated, numbing taste.

(Contd.)

Stramonium *(Datura stramonium)*	Stomata on the upper surface few, lower surface many, calcium oxalate in crystals, tirchomes conical, palisade one row with well marked crystal layers.
Henbane *(Hyoscyamus niger)*	Stomata on the upper surface few, lower surface many, cruciferous, calcium oxalate present, trichome large, ovoid well marked crystal layers in the mesophyll.
Henna *(Lawsonia inermis)*	Stomata Ranunculus type, trichomes absent, calcium oxalate in clusters, mesophyll differentiated epidermis over the veins is strongly straiated.

Some important plants with histological characters

(Flowers)

Name	Characters
	Floral Members
Clove *(Eugenia aromatica)*	Stalks contain calcium oxalate, epidermis of calyx is glabrous with stomata, corolla glabrous with oilglands and calcium crystals. Oil glands present in the apex of connective, pollen grain 15-20µ triangularly lenticular, few pericyclic fibres are special features, aromatic with pungent taste.
Lavender *(Lavendual officinalis)*	Calyx contains triangular trichome, corolla with labiate glandular trichomes, anther wall bears long trichomes, pollen grains spherical 38-42µ.
Arnica *(Arnica montana)*	Calyx modified with pappus bristles 5-6 cell wide, corolla ligulate, pollen grains spherical with 3 pores 40-52µ in diameter.

(Contd.)

Marigold	Corolla tube bears trichomes
Calendula officinale)	glandular and 120μ long.

Anatomical Study of
Root of *Rauwolfia serpentina*

MATERIAL SUPPLIED:	Root of *Rauwolfia serpentina* of family Apocynaceae.
PROCEDURE:	A T.S. of root was cut and permanent slide was prepared by using double stain with safranine and light green and was observed under the microscope.
OBSERVATION:	
External Morphology:	Roots sub-cylindrical, frequently curved, twisted, stout thick and of greyish yellow to brown colour with slightly wrinkled and rough surface, the intermediate colour being whitish grey.
Internal Morphology:	T.S. of root showed 8-10 layers of tubular cork cells with thicker walls, alternating with cells of larger and sometimes, smaller diameter. The intercellular space was lacking in secondary meristematic tissue. Phellogen was not distinquishable in the dry material. Primary cortex was crushed, secondary cortex containing parenchymatous cells heavily packed with starch grains. Secondary xylem formed major portion of the root consisting of wood parenchyma, trachea, and tracheid with pitted walls.

Anatomical Study of
Leaf of *Adhatoda vasica*

MATERIAL SUPPLIED:	Leaf of *Adhatoda vasica* of family Acanthaceae.
OBSERVATION:	
External Morphology:	Material was green in colour, upper surface less green than lower, simple, long, petiolate with prominent ridge at dorsal side of petiole, length 25.5 cm-12.5 cm and breadth

7.1 cm-3.4 cm, lanceolate, entire glabrous, acute at the base and slightly accuminate at the apex. Venation was unicostate reticulate. Odour slight, taste slightly bitter. Texture was leathery.

Internal Morphology: T.S of material showed wavy epidermis with thin outermost layer of cuticle. Epidermis scattered conical and glandular trichomes. Caryophyllaceous stomata were present on both surfaces but more on lower surface. 2 layers of palisade cells were present just beneath upper epidermis. Some cells contained cylindrical cysotoliths. Spongy parenchyma cells were present in 3-6 layers and arranged loosely. Midrib region showed 3-6 layers of chlorenchymatous tissue on dorsal and ventral side. Central region was occupied by 5 vascular bundles of which central one was the largest. Phloem was present on dorsal side and xylem was on the ventral side. Medullary rays transverse it. Ca-oxalate crystals were present in parenchymatous cortical cells.

Study of Stomatal Index

MATERIAL SUPPLIED: Leaf of *Adhatoda vasica*

PROCEDURE: A small piece of lamina between midrib and margin was taken. From this portion a thin transparent layer was peeled off from both upper and lower surface of leaf and then peelings were observed under microscope. Stomatal Index

$$S.I = \frac{S}{S + E} \times 100$$

where S = Total No. of Stomata / microscopic field of vision.

and E = Total No. of epidermal cells / microscopic field of vision.

OBSERVATION AND RESULT:
(a) Stomatal Index of upper surface

No. of observations	Total No. of stomatal microscopic field of vision	Total No. of epidermal cells/ microscopic field of vision	Mean total of stomata/micros: field of vision	Mean total of epidermal cell/ micros: field vision
1.	4	45		
2.	2	42	3	42.6
3.	3	41		

Therefore stomotal index of upper surface is

$$\frac{S}{S+E} \times 100 = \frac{3}{42.6+3} \times 100$$

$$= \frac{3 \times 100}{45.6}$$

$$= 6.5$$

(b) Stomatal Index of lower surface

No. of observations	Total No. of stomata/ microscopic field of vision (S)	Total No. of epidermal cells/ microscopic field of vision (E)	Mean total of stomata/ micros: field of vision.	Mean total of epidermal cells/ micros: field vision
1.	30	58		
2.	26	38	25.6	46.3
3.	21	43		

Therefore, stomatal index of lower surface is

$$\frac{S}{S+E} \times 100 = \frac{25.6}{25.6+46.3} \times 100$$

$$= \frac{25.6 \times 100}{71.9}$$

$$= 6.5$$

Rauwolfia serpentina

I. **Physical Observation:-**
   (a) **Colour** — Pale brownish yellow.
   (b) **Odour** — Slight.
   (c) **Taste** — Bitter.
   (d) **Fineness and degree of uniformity of particles:-** Moderate.
   (e) **Sensation of Smoothness** — Smooth.

II. **Microscopical Observations:**
   (a) **Starch Grains:** Abundant, mostly simple but compound granules were also found 2, 3/4 components, individual granules were spherical to irregular often large. 5-20μ, usually has a well-marked hilum in the form of a simple/radiate split.

   (b) **Calcium-oxalate crystals:** They were scattered and in small groups in some of the parenchymatous cells of phloem and medullary rays: They were irregularly prismatic and showed variation in size.

   (c) **Xylem fibres:** Numerous, irregular in shape, occur singly or in groups associated with vessels. Walls were lignified, moderately thickened and had small, slit shaped pits.

   (d) **Pericyclic fibres:** Very large, unlignified, with unevenly thickened walls and frequently showed elongated ovoid arrangement at one end.

   (c) **Vessels:** Single or in groups. They were fairly narrow with moderately thickened lignified walls and very small, numerous bordered pits. 36-54μ in diameter. They had a single perforation in the laeral walls at a short distance from the tapering ends.

   (d) **Stone cell:** None.

   (e) **Cork:** Many fragments of straitified reddish brown cork composed of polygonal cells. Some of which were lignified were observed.

   (f) **Parenchyma:-** Abundant fragments of lignified parenchyma filled with starch granules and composed of polygonal cells with moderately thickened walls. Xylem parenchyma was usually associated with tracheidal vessel.

Identifying Characters:
   (a) Leaf and flower elements absent.
   (b) Abundant parenchyma, starch numerous.

Root and Rhizome Drugs

(a) Stratified cork cells with lignified and unlignified bonds.
(b) Abundant parenchyma often filled with starch and ca-oxalate.
(c) Xylem elements lignified.
(d) Pericyclic fibres present.
(e) Some fibres with elongated ovoid enlargement near the end.
(f) Sclereids, phloem fibres and stone cells absent.

.... Root and Rhizome of **Rauwolfia serpentina.**

QUESTIONS

1. Today a paste containing bloodroot (*Sanguinaria canadensis*) which is used in conjunction with surgery to treat.
   (a) Skin Cancers   (b) Liver diseases
   (c) Kidney diseases   (d) Heart diseases

2. Resin from the *May apple* is still the preferred therapy for
   (a) Venereal warts   (b) Lung Cancer
   (b) Leprosy   (c) Tuberculosis

3. A balsam made by boiling *Sassafras* root (6 ounces), dogwood root (6 ounces) (till it be wasted to a pint) is used for
   (a) Curing cancer wounds (after operation)
   (b) Curing leprosy
   (c) Curing leucoderma
   (d) Curing wounds after operation

4. Drinking of *Sassafras* tea every morning is good for
   (a) Cancer patients   (b) Diabetic patients
   (c) High B.P. patients   (d) Tuberculosis patients

5. Which of the following are used to treat cancer
   (a) Seeds of common apricot (*Prunus armeniaca*)
   (b) Lactrile, a substance derived from an extract of apricot pits
   (c) Apricot Oil
   (d) Apple Seed Oil

6. Which of the following are cures for Cancer
   (a) Chaparral tea obtained from steeping leaves and stems of the creosote bush, *Larrea divaricata* in hot water.
   (b) CH-23, a secret remedy prepared from toxins contained in plants.
   (c) KC-555, derived from plants grown in Asia
   (d) Krebiozen, derived from extracts of the blood of horses previously injected with a sterile extract of *Actinomyces bovis*.

7. Gymnosperms which contain *anti-cancer* substances
   (a) *Juniperus virginiana* (Podophyllotoxin)
   (b) *Libocedrus decurrens* (deoxypodophyllotoxin)   ;
   (c) *Taxodium distichum* (taxodione and taxodene)
   (d) *Taxus baccata* (taxol)

8. A substance from the bacterium *Escherichia coli* which is a drug for acute lymphocytic leukemia.
   (a) Glutamine synthetase   (b) Glutamic dehydrogenase
   (c) Malate synthetase   (d) Asparaginase (Elspar)

9. Fungi which contain *anti-cancer* substances
   (a) *Amanita phalloides* (crude extracts); *Aspergillus fumigatus* (fumigillin)
   (b) *Boletus edulis* (fruiting body extracts); *Calvantia gigantea* (Calvacim); *Claviceps purpurea* (ergot)
   (c) *Penicillium sp. (mycophenolic acid); Poria corticola* (poricin)
   (d) All these

10. Which of the following terms contain anti-cancer substances?
    (a) *Pteridium aquilinum*
    (b) *Ophioglossum moluccanum*
    (c) *Polypodium leucotomos*
    (d) *Marsilea quadrifida*

11. Plants of India which contain *anti-cancer* substances
    (a) *Catharanthus (Vinca) roseus* Apocynaceae
    (b) *Podophyllum emodi*, Berberidaceae
    (c) *Stephania hernandifolia*, Menispermaceae
    (d) *Heliotropium indicum*, Boraginacae

12. *Cancer drug* from *Heliotropium indicum*, Boraginaceae
    (a) Indicine N-oxide   (b) Vinblastine sulphate
    (c) Podophyllotoxin   (d) Tetrandrine

13. Plants used as *panaceas* or universal remedies; used for stimulation, added energy, coughs, tuberculosis, nausea, diabetes, indigestion, diarrhoea, kidney degeneration, gout, rheumatism, suppurating, sores etc.
    (a) *Eleutherococcus senticosus*, Siberian ginseng, Araliaceae
    (b) *Panax ginseng*, Oriental ginseng, Araliaceae
    (c) *Panax quinquefolium*, American ginseng, Araliaceae
    (d) *Panax repans*, Chinese ginseng, Araliaceae

14. Which fungus is used in China as a tonic and stimulant for convalescents
    (a) *Agaricus campestris*   (b) *Psilocybe mexicana*
    (c) *Amanita muscaria*   (d) *Cordyceps sinensis*

15. Which are the compounds isolated from roots and leaves of *Ginseng?*
    (a) Panaxin acting as a stimulant for the midbrain, heart and vessels
    (b) Panax acid, as a stimulant for the heart and general metabolism
    (c) Panaquilin as a stimulant for internal secretions
    (d) Panacen and sapogenin volatile oils that stimulate the central nervous system; ginsenin that lowers blood sugar.

16. Which part of *Panax ginseng*, ginseng contain *anti-cancer* substances (steroids)
    (a) Root   (b) Leaves
    (c) Seeds   (d) Sperm

17. Plants which have at one time approached ginseng in local popularity?
    (a) *Hypoxis aurea*, Liliaceae (b) *Smilax* Liliaceae
    (c) *Corydalis* (Papaveraceae) (d) *Coptis teeta* (Ranunculaceae)

18. The anti-cancer drug *daunomycin* used in acute lymphocytic and granulocytic leukemia, is obtained from
    (a) *Streptomyces griseus*   (b) *Streptomyces scabies*
    (c) *Streptomyces peucetius*   (d) *Streptomyces venezuela*

19. The anti-cancer drug *streptozotocin*, used in malignant insulinoma, carcinoid, is obtained from
    (a) *Streptomyces griseus*   (b) *Streptomyces venezuela*
    (b) *Streptomyces aureofacieus* (c) *Streptomyces achromogenes*

20. The anti-cancer drug *adriamycin*, used in soft tissue, osteogenic and miscellaneous sarcomas, Hodgkin's disease, non-Hodgkin's lymphomas bronchogenic and breast carcinoma, is obtained from
    (a) *Streptomyces venezuela*
    (b) *Streptomyces peucetius* var *caesius*
    (c) *Streptomyces aureofaciuns*
    (d) *Streptomyces griseus*

21. Members of Piperaceae which contain *anti-cancer* substances?
    (a) *Piper nigrum*
    (b) *Piper longum*
    (c) *Piper brachystachum* (crotepoxide)
    (d) *Piper futokadzura P. Hookeri* (crotepoxide)

22. Members of Rosaceae which contain *anti-cancer* substance
    (a) *Amelanchier utachensis* June berry
    (b) *Rubus odoratus,* thimble berry
    (c) *Rosa damascana,* rose
    (d) *Pyrus malus,* apple

23. A foamy saponin or volatile oil to brighten stimulate and strengthen blonde hair, is made from
    (a) Chamomile (*Matricaria or Chamomilla*) + Yarrow (*Achillea millefolium*) 1:1
    (b) Rosemary, *Rosmarinus officinalis*
    (c) Garden sage, *Salvia officinalis*
    (d) *Asparagus africanus*

24. A suitable natural shampoo
    (a) Soapwort leaves *Saponaria officinalis* with powdered or extract of chamomile
    (b) *Canarium oleosum* leaves with chamomile
    (c) *Caryocar glarum* leaves with rosemary
    (d) *Yucca glauca* root with garden sage

25. An efficacious home remedy for dandruff
    (a) Infusion of rosemary mixed with a little borax
    (b) *Fallugia paradoxa* + borax
    (c) *Nardostachys jatamansi* + borax
    (d) *Pithecellobium bigeminum* + borax

26. A natural cure, particulartly for stomach or *intestinal cancer*
    (a) Eating of grapes 15 pounds per day for atleaset 6 weeks
    (b) Eating of 6 bananas per day for atleast 6 weeks
    (c) Eating of green vegetables for atleast 6 weeks
    (d) Eating of citrus fruits 6 per day, for atleast 6 weeks

27. "*Vervain (Verbena officinalis)* root was cut in half with one part hung around the patients's neck and the other hung to drug over a smouldering fire "This ancient Roman medicine was used to cure which disease?

(a) Cancer tumors (b) Nervous disorders
(b) Leucoderma (d) Jaundice

28. Eating of this cures uterine cancers, and obdominal tumours
    (a) Garlic (b) Onion
    (c) Turmeric (d) Ginger

29. The root sap of which plant was used for treatment of cancerous diseases
    (a) *Withania somnifera* (b) *Sanguinaria canadensis*
    (c) *Asparagus racemosus* (d) *Inula racemosa*

30. Paste of *bloodroot* extract, Zinc Chloride, flour and water the paste is smeared on a cloth or cotton and placed on the cancer tumour daily (if healthy tissue covered the tumor, it is eroded with nitric acid). When the tumor became entrusted, incisions are made about 1 to 1/2 inch apart and the paste is inserted into the cuts daily treatment 2 to 4 weeks. Who practise this technique to cure cancer?
    (a) Middelesex hospital, London
    (b) A.I.I.M.S, New Delhi
    (c) JIPMER, Pondicherry
    (c) VPCI, Delhi

31. Which plant is used to treat warts and nasal polyps, skin cancers in United States, and as a folk remedy in Russia
    (a) *Sanguinaria canadensis* (b) *Withania somnifera*
    (c) *Asparagus adscendens* (d) *Solanum tuberosum*

32. The resin of which plant was used in North America for the treatment of tumors, polyps unhealthy granulations and veneral- warts
    (a) *Podophyllum peltatum rhizome*
    (b) *Zingiber officinale rhizome*
    (c) *Curcuma longa, rhizome*
    (d) *Curcuma amada rhizome*

33. Iodine (used in treating carcinoma of the thyroid), phosphorus 32 (used in treating polycythemia vera, inhibiting the overproduction of red and white blood caells), gold 198 (used when cancer results in excessive fluid accumulation in the peritoneal cavity) are
    (a) Hormones (b) Radioactive isotopes
    (c) Antimetabolites (c) Alkylating agents

34. Which of the following hormones are effective in the treatment of breast carcinoma, prostrate carcinoma?
    (a) Diethylstilbestrol   (b) Ethenyl estradiol
    (b) Hydroxyprogesterone   (d) Megasterol acetate

35. *Androgens* effective in the treatment of breast cancer
    (a) Hydroxyprogesterone   (b) Megestrol aceta!
    (c) Testosterone propionate   (d) Testosterone enanthate,
        Testolactone

36. *Progestagens* used to treat metastatic and recurent endometrical carcinoma
    (a) Testolactone   (b) Hydroxy Progesterone
    (b) Megestrol acetate   (d) Testosterone priopontate

37. *Vincristine Sulphate* (Oncovin) obtained fron (*Vinca rosea*) is used in
    (a) Hodgkin's disease   (b) Choriocarcinoma
    (c) Acute leukemia in Children (d) Testicular tumours

38. Drugs of plant origin used to treat testicular tumours
    (a) Dactinomycin   (b) Mithramycin
    (c) Methothrexate   (d) Chlorambucil

39. Drugs of plnat origin used to treat *Hodgkin's disease* (a type of cancer)
    (a) Vincristine   (b) Prednisone, Procarbazine
    (c) Bleomycin   (d) Nitrogen mustard

40. Drugs of plant origin used to treat *Wilm's tumor*
    (a) Vincristine   (b) Dactinomycin
    (c) Surgery   (d) Radiotherapy

41. Drugs of plant origin used to treat acute lymphocytic leukemia
    (a) Vincristine   (b) Prednisone
    (c) Daunomycin   (d) Nitrogen mustard

42. Match the following anti-cancer drugs and the organisers from which these are extracted.
    (a) Dactinomycin   1. *Streptomyces parvulpus*
    (b) Mithramycin   2. *Streptomyces plicatus*
    (c) Bleomycin sulphate   3. *Streptomyces verticillatus*
    (d) Adramycin   4. *Streptomyces peucetius var vaesius*

43. Match the following:

    (a) Datctinomycin
    (b) Mithramycin

    (c) Steptozotocin

    (d) Blemycin sulphate

    1. *Binds directly to DNA*
    2. *Inhibit ; the synthesis of RNA*
    3. *Used against carcinoid tumours of the appendix*
    4. *Used against squamous cell carcinomas in the head and secretions.*

44. Plant families with species most active against cancer
    (a) Apocynaeae, Celastraceae (b) Magnoliaceae, Rutaceae
    (c) Simaroubaceae   (d) Thymelaeaceae

45. "Once inside the body, apricot pits breakdown into several components. When it comes into contact with an enzyme common to tumour cells, β-glycuronidase, cynide is relesed, which chokes off tumor cells having the healthy cells surrounding the growth untouched "which therapy is based on this concept
    (a) Radioactive isotopes for curing cancer
    (b) Chemotherapy for curing cancer
    (c) Neutron therapy for curing cancer
    (d) Lactrile therapy for curing cancer

46. *Nitrogen mustard* (mustine hydrochloride) is able to kill malignant cells during all phases of their cycle bty combining chemicallyo with
    (a) Necleic acids   (b) Proteins
    (c) Carbohydrates   (d) Aminoacids

47. *Alkylating agest* used against Hodgkin's disease and other lymphomas. lymphocytic leukemia, and certain solid cancers.
    (a) Mechlorethamine (Mustargen), Thiotepa, Chloramkucil
    (b) Cyclophosphamide, Triethylene melamine,
    (c) Melphalan, Busulfan
    (d) All these

48. *Antimetabolites* (which kill cells at the time of DNA synthesis in prepartion for cell division, either by depriving the cell of vital substrates, necessary for DNA synthesis or by being incorporated into DNA synthesis or by being incor-porated into DNA as gradulent precursors used in cancer treatment

(a) Methotrexater Mercaptopurine, Thioguanine, Fluorouracil, Cytarabine

(b) Prednisone, Ethinyl estradiol, Testosterone propionate

(c) Testolactone, Hydroxyprogesterone, Megastrol acetate, Testosterone Propionate

(d) Testosterone enanthate Diethylstilbestrol

49. *Colchicine alkaloid* obtained from the autumn crocus, *Colchicum autumnale* acts by

(a) Disrupting the spindle mechanism during mitosis thereby blocking cell division

(b) Disrupting meiotic cell division

(c) Causing non-stop cell divisions

(d) Disrupting the movement of chromosomes in anaphase of mitosis

50. Crude extract of this plant drastically reduced white blood cell counts, especially the granulocytes and profoundly depressed bone marrow activity in rats.

(a) *Vinca rosea,*   (b) *Heliotropium indicum*

(c) *Sanguinaria canadensis*   (d) *Withania somnifera*

51. *Vincolucoblastine, leurocristine* (now considered the drug of choice) which induce remissions in childhood leukemia are obtained from

(a) *Vinca rosea,*   (b) *Heliotropium indicum*

(c) *Sanguinaria canadensis*   (d) *Withania somnifera*

52. *Vincoblastine sulphate* (Velbaw) obtained from *Vinca rosea* is particularly usefull in

(a) Hodgkin's disease   (b) Choriocarcinoma

(c) Other neoplasms   (d) All these

53. A common craze for *mehandi (henna)* in England is due to its effective treatment for conditioning hair and as a powerfull anti-dandruff agent, Mehandi is obtained from

(a) *Symplocos recemosa,* Symplocaceae

(b) *Madhuca indica,* Sapotacae

(c) *Lawsonia inermis,* Lythraceae

(d) *Coptis teeta,* Ranunculaceae

54. Roots of which of the following plants contain *diosgenin* which forms cortisone used for oral contraceptive.
    (a) *Balanites aegyptiaca*, Simarubaceae
    (b) *Solanum surattense*, Solanaceae
    (c) *Sida cordifolia*, Malvaceae
    (d) *Withania somnifera*, Solanaceae

55. A medicinal plant common in marshy grounds, throughout India, very common in Hardwar swamps
    (a) *Prosopis spicigera*, Mimosaceae
    (b) *Bacopa monieria*, Scrophulariaceae
    (c) *Acacia catechu*, Mimosaceae
    (d) *Ferula foetida*, Umbelliferae

56. In India *Ferula narthex* is found in
    (a) Dry and barren tracts of Himachal
    (b) Kashmir   (c) Kumaon westwards
    (d) Aravalli mountain ranges

57. The gum-resin *guggulu* obtained from *Commiphora mukul* Burseraceae is useful for
    (a) Heart troubles
    (b) Stopes sclerotosis, coronary-thrombosis and coronary artery troubles
    (c) Anti-arthritis
    (d) All these

58. Which of the following is wrong; Seed oil of *Cannabis sativa. Bhang* is used as
    (a) Luminant   (b) Paints and Varnishes
    (c) Soaps   (d) Cooking medium

59. Turkish intoxicating preparation, *hashish*, is made from which part of the bhang (Indian hemp) plant?
    (a) Leaves   (b) Flowering tops
    (c) Seeds   (d) Seed husk

60. Egyptian intoxicating preparation from the *bhang* plant is made from
    (a) Leaves   (b) Flowering tops
    (c) Sees   (d) Seed husk

61. The oil extracted from the seeds of *Carallia brachiata* Karalli, Rhizophoraceae is used as
    (a) Cooking medium   (b) Cheese making
    (c) Chocolates   (d) Sweets

62. A common house-hold remedy for *stomach trouble*
    (a) Prasarini, *Paederia scandens*, Rubiaceae
    (b) Prisniparni, *Uvaria lagopodies*, Fabaceae
    (c) Priyange, *Aglaia roxburghiana*, Meliaceae
    (d) Pudina, *Mentha arvensis*, Labiatae

63. "Tender shoots are eaten as pot-herb. Root powder mixed with *mamira* is used in eye diseases.
    (a) *Tribulus terrestis*, Zygophyllaceae
    (b) *Tephrosia purpurea*, Fabaceae
    (c) *Tridax procumbens*, Asteraceae
    (d) *Boerhaavia diffusa*, Nyctaginaceae

64. Commercial *asafoetida* is adultered with
    (a) Gum arabic, other gum-resins
    (b) Rosin gypsum, red clay, chalk
    (c) Berley, wheat-flower slices of potatoes
    (d) All these

65. Which of the follwoing are wrong
    (a) Banda mace is considered to be the finest. It has a bright orange colour and fine aroma
    (b) Java estate mace is golden yellow, interspersed with brilliant crimson streaks like Banda mace. It is free from insect infestation.
    (c) Siauw mace is of lighter colour than Banda mace and contains less volatile oil.
    (d) Mace is the fruit of *Myristica fragrans*, jatiphal.

66. *Papua mace* (Macassar mace) is obtained from
    (a) *Myristica fragrans*   (b) *Myristica argentica*
    (c) *Myristica malabarica*   (d) *All these*

67. *Bombay mace* or wild mace is obtained from
    (a) *Myristica fragrans*   (b) *Myristica argentica*
    (c) *Myristica malabarica*   (d) All these

68. *Piney oil* (Dil Oil) used in soap making and as a luminant is obtained from seeds of
    (a) *Calophyllum inophyllum*, Guttiferae
    (b) *Argemone mexicana*, Papaveraceae
    (c) *Cannabis sativa*, Cannabinceae
    (d) *Papaver somniferim*, Papaveraceae

69. Members of Malvaceae used as *edible greens*
    (a) *Althaea officinalis (marsh mallow); Sida veronicaefolia (phiuli)*
    (b) *Hibiscus surattensis (chirval), Pavonia odorata*
    (c) *Malva parviflora* (panirak), *Malva roundifolia* (Khubasi), *Malva sylvestris* (Kunzi, gulkhair), *Malva verticillata*
    (d) All these

70. Which of the following are correct
    (a) Hingra is the exudate of *Ferula foetida*
    (b) Hings is the exudate of *Ferula asafoetida*
    (c) Banthani hing is a compounded asafoetida composed of one or more varieties of asafoetida (Irani or Pathani hing or both)
    (d) All these

71. Which factors influence the Quality and flavour of *asafoetida?*
    (a) Part of the plant from which prepared
    (b) The season of collection
    (c) The method of preparation
    (d) The nature and degree of adulterant

72. *Asafoetida* (hing or hingra) is a
    (a) Germ   (b) Resin
    (c) Essential Oil   (d) Oleogum resin

73. Which of the following are correct
    (a) Bitter asafoetida is obtained from the cutting of the plant root (tap root).
    (b) Sweet asfoetida is obtained from the horizontal cutting of the stem.
    (c) Among the Irani and Pathani hing, Hadda variety is the most priced and the strongest.
    (d) Asafoetida is exuded from the living rhizome of the plant.

74. What is the extent of *Saffaron* cultivation in India (in acres)?
    (a) 3350   (b) 33500

    (c) 335000   (d) 3350000

75. Areas in which *saffron* is cultivated in India?
    (a) Kisthwar region of Jammu
    (b) Pampore near Srinagar
    (c) Gangotri in the Himalayas
    (d) Shimla region of Himalayas

76. India imports *Saffron* from
    (a) Spain   (b) France
    (c) Portugal   (d) Mexico

77. The flowering period of *saffron* (*Crocus sativus*, Iridaceae)
    (a) Middle or late January to first or second seek of March
    (b) Late March to Middle of July
    (c) Late July to late August
    (d) Middle or late October to first or second week of November

78. Adulterants of true *saffron* are
    (a) Meadow saffron, *Colchicum autumnale*, Liliaceae
    (b) Bastard saffron, *Carthamus tinctorius*, Compositae
    (c) Coal tar dyes, corn silk, *Calendula* sp.
    (d) All theese

79. Foods in which *saffron* is used
    (a) Spanish rice specialities
    (b) French fish preparations
    (c) Used in fine bread in Scandinavia
    (d) Used in sweets in India

80. *Sage* is the dried leaf of
    (a) *Salvia officinalis*, Labiatae
    (b) *Satureia hortensis* Labiatae
    (c) *Thymus vulgaris*, Labiatae
    (d) *Coleus amboinicus* Labiatae

81. Mangroves with *edible fruits*
    (a) *Rhizophora mucronata*   (b) *Sonneretia acida*
    (c) *Firmiana colorata* ·   (d) *Sterculia guttata*

82. Mangroves with *edible greens*
    (a) *Salicornia brachiata*   (b) *Salsola baryosma Kali*
    (c) *Firmiana colorata*   (d) *Avicennia officinalis*

83. What are the economic uses of *sundri (Heritiera minor, Sterculiaceae)*, a mangrove plant with pneumatophores.
    (a) Sundri charcoal is specially used for gun powder
    (b) Wood is used as pile wood, pit props boat making, card axles, agricultural implements, railway keys.
    (c) Leaves are used in tanning
    (d) Bark is used in tanning

84. What are the economic users of *Rhizophora mucronata*, bhora, Kandal, rai Rhizophoraceae) a mangrove plant:
    (a) Wood is valuable as fuel and for making charcoal
    (b) Bark contains tannin useful for tanning leather
    (c) Bark is used for dyeing leather brown for toughening fishing lines and ropes
    (d) The mature fruit is sweet; edible. A Light wine is prepared from the juices of the fruit.

85. The seeds of which of the following grasses (members of Graminae) are used as *scarcity or famine foods*
    (a) *Bambusa bambos; Brachiaria deflexa, Brachiaria reptans*
    (b) *Cenchrus biflorus, Cenchrus prieurie: Chrysopogon fulvus* goria, gogar;
    (c) *Dactyloctenium aegyptium* makra;, *Dendrocalamus strictus* banskaban; *Echinochloa colonum,* Sawan; *Echinochloa crusgalli* Sawan; *Elyonurus hirsutus, Eragrostis tremula* Dhot-Phulia;
    (d) *Hygroryza aristata, Ischaemum rugosum, Oryza rufipogon, Sacciolepis interrupta, Setaria glauca* Bandra; *Setaria pallidefusca Urochola panicoides, Zizania latifolia*

86. The seed flour of which of the following is a *substitute for arrowroot*
    (a) *Euryale ferox,* gorgan nut, makhana
    (b) *Nelumbo nucifera,* Kamal
    (c) *Nymphaea nouchali,* Kamal Kakri
    (d) *Nymphaea tetrasgona*

87. The fruits of which of the following cucurbits are used as *scarcity or famine foods?*
    (a) *Kedrostis prostrata, Trichosanthes dioica palwal*
    (b) *Coccinea cordifolia, Kundri; Trichosanthes cucumerina, Jangli chachind*
    (c) *Cucumis melo*

(d) *Melotria heterophylla* Kundri; *Momordica balsamina, Mikha, M. charantia, Jungli Karela; M. cochinchinensis, Kokrol, M. dioica, Kakawra*

88. *Kekuna Oil* obtained from the edible nut of *Aleurites moluccana* Euphorbiaceae is used in
    (a) Paint, varnish industries
    (b) As a hair tonic
    (c) Cooling purposes
    (d) For making candles

89. Which of the following trees yield *oils*
    (a) *Argemone mexicana, Artemisia absinthium, Azadirachta indica, Balanites aegyptiaca, Berberis aristata, Bombax malabaricum*
    (b) *Buchanania lanzan, Calophyllum inophyllum, Cannabis sativa, Carallia brachiata,Carthaus olycantha, Carthamus tinctorius, Cedurs deodara, Ceiba pentandra*
    (c) *Cinnamomum tamala, Cocos nucifera, Diplokena butyracea, Garcinia indica, Garcinia morella, Jatropha curcas*
    (d) *Mimusops elengi, Moringa oleifera, Palaquium ellipticum, Pongamia pinnata, Ricinus communis, Schleichera oleosa.*

90. *Rogherun oil*, very much used by the peshawari artizan for the manufacutre of Afridi wax cloth; oil clothes, Tarpaulins and tent cloth:used for greasing well ropes, well buckets and leather articles used for drawing water from wells is obtained from the seeds of
    (a) *Carthamus oxycantha*, Kantiari, Compositae
    (b) *Carthamus tinctorius*, Kusumba, Compositae
    (c) *Helianthus annus*, Surajmukhi, Compositae
    (d) *Lactuca serriola* Kahu, Compositae

91. Which of the following *oil* is used in food, for pressurings leather goods and in white paints
    (a) Safflower oil
    (b) Poli Oil
    (c) Roghien Oil
    (d) Kikuna Oil

92. *Phulwara Butter*, an edible vetable butter used as a substitute for ghee and also for cocoa butter is obtained from seeds of
    (a) *Achras sapota*, Sapodilla, Sapotaceae
    (b) *Sideroxylon indicerm*, Sapotaceae
    (c) *Bassia latifolia*, Mahua, Sapotaceae
    (d) *Diploknema butyracea*, phulal, Sapotaceae

93. The flowers of which of the following plants contain sugars and are used in the manufacture of gur-like preparations and spritious liquors
    (a) *Diploknema butyracea*, Phulel (Sapotaceae)
    (b) *Madhuca indica*, Mowra (Sapotaceae)
    (c) *Madhuca longifolia* mawra (Sapotaceae
    (d) All these

94. The gum resin *gamboge* of commerce is obtained form
    (a) *Garcinia indica*, Kokam, Guttiferae
    (b) *Garcinia morella*, tamal, Guttiferae
    (c) *Mimusops hexandra*, guttapercha, Sapotaceae
    (d) *Siderolylon indiceum*, iron wood, Sapotaceae

95. *Bimli jute* fibre is obtained from
    (a) *Hibiscus cannabinus*   (b) *Hibiscus rosa -sinensis*
    (c) *Hibiscus ficulneus*   (d) *Hibiscus collinus*

96. Economic use of charoli, *Chironji, Buchannia Lanzan,* Anacardiaceae are
    (a) Seeds are used in confectionery. Fruit is an important article of food.
    (b) Bark is used in tanning; it yields a natural varnish
    (c) Gum is used for dressing textiles, printing cloth and dyeing
    (d) Wood is for door and window frames; match boxes (not match sticks)

97. Phytachemagglutinin used in passive immunotherapy for cancer is obtained from
    (a) Kidney bean, *Phaseolus vulgaris*
    (b) Red gram, *Cajanus cajan*
    (c) Green gram, *Phaseolus aureus*
    (d) Black gram, *Phaseolus mungo*

98. *Mutagens* derived from plant lectius (used in passive immunotherapy for cancer) are obtained from
    (a) *Phytolacca americana* pokeweed mitogen
    (b) *Wisteria floribunda*
    (c) *Canavalia ensiformis*, Concanavalin
    (d) *Lathyrus odoratus*

99. Members of Apocynaceae which contains *anti-cancer* substances
    (a) *Catharanthus lanceus (leurosine)*
    (b) *Ochrosia elliptica   O. moorei & O. poweri (ellipticine)*
    (c) *Apocynum cannabinum (apocannoside, cymarium)*
    (d) *Bleekeria sp.* (ellipticina); *Excavation coccinea* (ellipticine)

100. Anti-Cancer drugs obtained from *Colchium autumnale* Liliaceae
    (a) Demecolcine   (b) Colchicine
    (c) Tetrandrine   (d) Thalicarpine

101. *Spearmint,* pahari pudiana (dried leaves are used as a spice)
    (a) *Mentha arvensis,* Labiatae
    (b) *Mentha piperita,* Labiatae
    (c) *Mentha arvensis var piperascens,* Labiatae
    (d) *Mentha spicata* Labiatae

102. Brown mustard is
    (a) *Brassica nigra,* Crucifere
    (b) *Brassica junca,* Crucifeae
    (c) *Brassica alba,* Cruciferae
    (d) *Brassica campestris var toria,* Crucifeae

103. What are the economic users of *long pepper,* pipli *Piper lonigum,* Piperaceae
    (a) Fruits used in pickles and preserves
    (b) Antitubercular activity against *Mycobacterium tuberculosis*
    (c) Dried stems (piplamul) are used in medicine against couph, bronchitius, asthma
    (d) In Andaman Leaves are chewed; root is used to permanent rice beer

104. *Long pepper* leaves and fruits are active against
    (a) *Mycobacterium tuberculosis*
    (b) *Micrococcus phygenes*
    (c) *Escherichia coli*
    (d) All these bacteria

105. What are the economic uses of *poppy seeds (Papaver somniferum* Papaveraceae)
    (a) Seeds are considered nutritive and are used in breads, curriees, sweets and confectionery

(b) Seeds are demulcent used as an emollient

(c) Specific against obstinate constipation and catarh of the bladder

(d) Used in the production of lecithin

106. In India, *Baby's tonic* and anti-diarrhotic and dysenteric medicines like Gripe-water and ghuttis are prepared from which part of rhubarb, rewandichini (*Rheum emodi*, Polygonaceae)
    (a) Roots   (b) Leaves
    (c) Stem   (d) Seeds

107. Which of the following plants contain *diosgenin* in leaves, stem and fruits (diosgenin is a source for cortisone and sex hormones)
    (a) *Solanum tuberosum*, Alu
    (b) *Solanum, nigrum*
    (c) *Solanum melongena*, Baigan
    (d) *Solanum indicum*, Barikaeri

108. *Cubib cigarettes* (Piper cubeba, Kabeb chini) are smoked to relieve
    (a) Headache   (b) Asthma
    (c) Hay Fever   (d) Boils in nose

109. Which variety of Khadin is found in Northern India?
    (a) *Acacia sundra*   (b) *Acacia catechu var typica*
    (c) *Acacia catechunoides*   (d) All these

110. What is the economic use of *catechu* obtained from *Acacia catechu*?
    (a) Cleaning the petrol-pipes
    (b) Descaling of boiler
    (c) Colouring sail clothes and marine cordages
    (d) A remedy in relaxed throat.

111. *Tamarind* (imli) fruit contains
    (a) Tartaric acid 5 per cent, citric acid 4 per cent
    (b) Malic acid, Acetic acid, gum Pectin
    (c) Potassium tartrate 8 per cent
    (d) Sugar 25-40 per cent

112. *Tamarind* (imli) seeds contains mainly
   (a) Starch and pectin   (b) Sugar and gum
   (c) Organis acids and pectin (d) Tartaric acid

113. In the Northern Indian markets which plant/s are sold as a *mlavetas.*
   (a) Dried leaf - stalk of rhubarb, *Rheum emodi*
   (b) Acidic citrus fruits
   (c) Acidic fruits and leaves of *Garcinia pedunculata*, Guttifeae
   (d) All these

114. What are the economic uses of *Garcinia pediculata* in India
   (a) Leaves are used in cooking fish and tendering meat
   (b) Fruit makes refreshing sweet drink
   (c) Considered good for cold, cough and hiccough
   (d) Useful in loss of appetite, indigestion, constipation, heart weakness and in rheumatic troubles.

115. Which part of *Kokam Tree* (*Garcinia indica*) is used as a condiment to given an acid flavour to curries and also for preparing cooling syrups during hot months.
   (a) Leaves   (b) Flowers
   (c) Roots   (d) Fruits

116. *Stone leek*, used for flouring farely diets of eastern people is
   (a) *Allium sativum Liliaceae*
   (b) *Allium cepa, Liliaceae*
   (c) *Allium fistulosum, Liliaceae*
   (d) *Asparagus sarmentosus*, Liliaceae

117. Botaonical name and family of *lovage*, the roots, seeds and leaves of which are used for flavouring foods; seeds are used for flavouring confectionery
   (a) *Majorana hortensis*, Labiatae
   (b) *Origanum vulgare*, Labiatae
   (c) *Coriandrum sativum*, Umbellifeae
   (d) *Levisticum officinale*, Umbelliferae

118. *Saffron* is obtained from
   (a) *Carthamus tinctorius*, Compositae
   (b) *Colchicum autuynnale*, Liliaceae

(c) *Butea monosperma*, Papilionaceae

(d) *Crocus sativus*, Iridaceae

119. *Shahi Saffron* (first grade saffron) is obtained from which part of saffron plant
    (a) Dried stigmas of flowers
    (b) Dried petals of flowers
    (c) Dried stamens of flowers
    (d) Dried bulbs

120. Saffron when pounded with ghee, is reported to be very effective in curing
    (a) Diabetes
    (b) Malaria
    (c) Cancer
    (d) Skin diseases

121. Saffron soaked overring in water and used with honey, is useful in curing
    (a) Urine troubles
    (b) Liver disease
    (c) Feavers
    (d) Lung troubles

122. Shallot bulbs used as a condiment are obtained from
    (a) *Allium ascalonicum*, Liliaceae
    (b) *Allium sativum*, Liliaceae
    (c) *Allium cepa*, Liliaceae
    (d) *Allium fisfulosum*, Liliaceae

123. In Ghana, *Shallot bulbs* are gound and rubbed on the skins of children to cure which disease? Shallout is mixed with palm vine and large pepper and heated in the sun, the mixture is used to cure which disease.
    (a) Diabetes
    (b) Fever
    (c) Nervous debility
    (d) Skin diseases

124. *Star-anise* is the dried, star -shaped fruit derived from
    (a) *Pimpinella anisum*, Umbelliferae
    (b) *Liriodendron tulifera*, Magnoliaceae
    (c) *Michelia champaca*, Magnoliaceae
    (d) *Illicium verum*, Magnoliaceae

125. Which country prepares medicnial tea from the leaves of *star-anise*? who believe that 1 or 2 carpels of star anise when added to chicken which is to be roasted improve its flavour tremendously?

(a) India   (b) China

(c) Ghana   (d) Egypt

126. Which of the following members of Amaranthaceae are used as *Scarcity or Fanine foods*?

   (a) *Achyranthus aspera, Aerva lanata*

   (b) *Alternanthera sessilis, Arthocnemum indicum, Alternanthera triandra,*

   (c) *Amarnthus spinosus, Amaranthus tricolor, A. viridis, A. blifum*

   (d) *Celosia argentea, Digera arvensis, Nothosaerva brachiata, Roditia amherstiana*

127. Which members of Gramineae are used as *edible greens?*

   (a) Young shoots of *Bambusa tulda*

   (b) Young shoots of *Dendrocalamus hamiltonii*

   (c) Young shoots of *Cynodon dactylon*

   (d) Young shoots of *Eragrostis ciliaris*

128. *Allspice* comprises the dried unripe berries which are nearly globular, Z-7 mm in diameter, with a somewhat rough surface and a reddish brown colour. Allspice is obtained from

   (a) *Pimenta officinalis* Myrtaceae

   (b) *Syzygium aromaticum,* Myrtaceae

   (c) *Melaeuca leucodendron* Myrtaceae

   (d) *Barringtonia acutangula,* Myrtaceae

129. Which spice is used to flavour French-type alcoholic liquors and especially in *gin absenthe*

   (a) *Apium root*   (b) *Pimpinella root*

   (c) *Carum root*   (d) *Angelica root*

130. *Juniper* berries is largely used in

   (a) Flavouring gin, liquor and cordials

   (b) Treatment of gonorrhoea

   (c) Disorders of Urino-genital treat

   (d) Flavouring food products

131. Which of the following Solanums have edible fruits?

   (a) *Solanum indicum, Birhatta*

   (b) *Solanum torvum, tit-began*

(c) *Solanum spirate, Solanum rurzil*

(d) *Solanum incanum, Solanum erianthemum*

132. Which of the following are mainly used as scarcity or famine foods?

    (a) *Physalis minima*, tulatipati, ripe berries

    (b) Podophyllum hexandrum rapra, ripe berries

    (c) *Solanum stramonifolium*, ripe berries

    (d) *Toddalia asiatica* Kanj fruit puls

133. Which part *Tacca leontopetaloides*, East Indian arrowroot, diva yield starch?

    (a) Roots   (b) Rhizome

    (c) Aerial Stem   (d) Leaves

134. Economic importance of *Eriosma chinease*, Kondan; *Potentilla mooniara, Moghania vestita, Vigna cayensis*, halunda

    (a) Roots   (b) Rhizome

    (c) Aerial stem   (d) Leaves

135. Which of the following *ferns* fronds when yound in folded state are used as vegetables in the Himalayas:

    (a) *Petridium aquilinum*   (b) *Pleopetis insignis*

    (c) *Alsophila plecipens*   (d) *Nephrodium multicaudatum*

136. Which of the following members of compositee are used as *edible greens*?

    (a) *Asteracantha longibolie, Cichorium intybus, Scorzonera* sp.

    (b) *Cirsium lipstlyi, Emilia sonchifolia, Sonchus oberaceus*

    (c) *Enhydra fluctuans, Lactuca scariola, Taraxacum officinale*

    (d) *Launaea nudicalis, Pieris hieraciorides, Vernonia cinerea*

137. Economic uses of *tamarind (Tamarindus indica)* chinch, imli) seed oil are

    (a) Varnish for wooden furniture

    (b) Varnish for painting images and idols

    (c) Varnish for automobiles

    (d) Varnish for oil-cloth

138. *Misri lei*, a mnnan found on twigs of *Tamarix aphylla* karot, hal, jhau, punctured by insects, is used for

    (a) Tanning leather   (b) Dyeing fabrics

    (c) Fermenting sugar   (d) Adulterating sugar

139. Galls formed on flowers of *Tamarix dioica* Roxle, jhau, attacked by insects are used for
     (a) Tanning   (b) Dyeing
     (c) Tanning and Dyeing   (d) Adultering sugar

140. *Gazanbeen* an exudate from insect puncutres on the stem and branches of *Tamarix troupie* Hole. Jhan is a
     (a) Gem   (b) Oleo resin
     (c) Resing   (d) Manna

141. Alkaloid *trigonelline* is present in the seeds of
     (a) Dhania   (b) Methi
     (c) Ajwain   (d) Zeera

142. *Malabar Tallow* or piney tallow a vegetable butter used in confectionery; in the manufacture of soaps and candles is obtained from
     (a) *Vateria indica*, dhup maram
     (b) *Viloa odorata*, banaf shah
     (c) *Terminalia catappa*, Jungli badam
     (d) *Terminalia chebula*, harra

143. What is the common economic use of fruits and fruit ash of *Adansonia digitata* gorakh, amli, leaves of *Ahatoda vasica*, Vasaka Oil Cake of *Aleurites moluccana*, Bengal Walnut, *Argemone mexicana*, Bharbandi, *Azadirachta indica*, neem; leaves of bamboo.
     (a) Edible foods   (b) Tannins
     (c) Dyes   (d) Fertilizer

144. What is the common economic use of oil cake of *Madhuca indica*, Mahua; *Madhuca longifolia*, mahua, *Mallotus philippinensis*, Kanda; *Moringa oleifera*, Mungna; *Pongamia pinnata*, Karanj.
     (a) Dyes   (b) Tannins
     (c) Gums   (d) Fertilizer

145. Dried leaves and branches of *Pogostemon heyneanus*, Labiatae form
     (a) Patchouli of commerce
     (b) Chandni; tagara of commerce
     (c) Pachuk of commerce
     (d) Petitgrain of commerce

146. *Pachuk* of commerce an essential oil used in the preparation of rich perfumes and hair oils is obtained from which part of the plant *Saussurea lappa* of composit ie?
    (a) Flowers   (b) Leaves
    (c) Fruits   (d) Roots

147. In folds of shawls and woolen clothes, which roots are kept to protect them from insects and to impart characteristic perfume.
    (a) Pachuk   (b) Arua
    (c) Maha nim   (d) Nair

148. The leaves of which plant yield a perfume used as a substitute for petitgrain oil?
    (a) Chandni, *Tabernaemontana coronaria*
    (b) Chandan, *Santalum album*
    (c) Ain, *Terminalia tomentosa*
    (d) Nair, *Skimmia laureola*, Rutaceae

149. The blood root plant *Sanguinaria canadensis* which contains anti-cancer drugs sanguinarine and chelergthrine, belongs to the angiosperm family
    (a) Magnoliaceae   (b) Menispermacae
    (c) Asteraceae   (d) Papaveraceae

150. Anti - cancer susbstance containing plants from Solanaceae
    (a) *Withania coagulans, W. somnifera* (withanolids)
    (b) *Solanum dulcamara* (β -solamarine)
    (c) *Solanum tripartitum* (*Solapalmitine solapalmitinine*)
    (d) *Jaborosa integrifolia* (Jaborosolides)

151. Which of the following plants are used as insecticides
    (a) Seeds of *Ipomaea quamoclitf, Jacquemontia tamnifolia*, Convolvulaceae
    (b) Roots of *Dolichos pseudopachyrhizus, Lonchocarpus nocore*, Fabaceae
    (c) Fruit powder of *Melia azedarach*, Meliaceae
    (d) Leaf dust of *Nicotiana tabacum N. rustica*

152. The orchids -*Anoctochilus, Erythrodes, Goodyera, Haemaria, Macodes, Zeuxine* are commonly known as
    (a) Golden butterfly orchids (b) Lady slippers
    (c) Dove orchids   (d) Jewel orchids

153. Water-chestnut Singhara *Trapa bispinosa, Trapa quadrispinosn* are found mainly in
    (a) Punjab
    (b) Jammu and Kashmir
    (c) Tamil Nadu and in parts of Maharashtra
    (d) Bihar and Uttar Pradesh

154. *Tabashir or Banslochan* a mineral or silicous concretion, of various shades of brown colour is found in which part of the bamboo plant?
    (a) Leaves   (b) Shoots
    (c) Roots   (d) Culms

155. Which of the following are present in *Tabashir or Bansalochan*?
    (a) Nuclease   (b) Urease
    (c) Proteolytic enzymes (d) Cholin, Betain

156. *Giant bamboo (Dendrocalamus giganteus)* the tallest of bamboos, grows to which height (in centi meters) in a period of 24 hours?
    (a) 1   (b) 2
    (c) 7.5   (d) 35-40

157. *Golden bamboo* which has beautiful yellow and green striped culms is
    (a) *Bambusa vulgaris*   (b) *Bambusa tulda*
    (c) *Bambusa bambos*   (d) *Bambusa arundinacea*

158. *Cymbidium elegans*, a rare epiphytic orchid is native to
    (a) Subtropical Himalayas, Khasi Hills, Manipur hills
    (b) Western Ghats
    (c) Aravalli mountain range
    (d) Deccan

159. *Vanda coerulea* (blue orchid) is native to
    (a) Khasi Hills   (b) Manipur Hills
    (c) Nilgiri Hills   (d) Annamali Hills

160. The blue flower of the blue orchid blooms during
    (a) September to December (b) Jan to March
    (c) March to July   (d) July to August

161. *Indian Cherry* or Sebesten, widely grown in India and Sri
     Lanka is
     (a) *Cordia dichotoma*, lasora, Boraginaceae
     (b) *Cordia crenata*, gondi, Boraginaceae
     (c) *Cordia vestita*, godela Boraginaceae
     (d) All type

162. How many anthers are present in the male and imperfect
     hermaphrodite flowers of *Litchi chinensis*?
     (a) 6   (b) 9
     (c) 69   (d) Zero

163. *Litchi* is the backbone of which industry in and around
     Muzaffarpur (Bihar)
     (a) Fruit Jam   (b) Silk
     (c) Pickles   (d) Bee- Keeping

164. Which bee can pollinate the numerous flowers of *Litchi*
     effectively and successfully?
     (a) *Apis cerana*   (b) *Apis cerana - indica*
     (c) *Apis florea*   (d) *Apis dorsata*

165. Marginal Scorching of older leaves and lack of shine and
     lustre in apple fruits; June drop of apple fruits is due to the
     deficiency of
     (a) Calcium   (b) Zinc
     (c) Potassium   (d) Boron

166. Small bitter gourd, *Momordica dioica* Kakrol (diploid variety
     2n-28) grows wild in
     (a) Hills of Raj Mahal, Hazaribagh and Rajgir in Bihar
     (b) Hilly regions of Pune district of Maharashtra
     (c) Western Rajasthan desert
     (d) All these areas

167. Small bitter gourd, *Momordica dioica* (tetraploid 4n = 56)
     grows wild in
     (a) Western Rajasthan desert
     (b) Hilly regions of Pune district of Maharashtra
     (c) Khasi and Jaintia hill of Assam and Darjeeling
     (d) Hazaribagh in Bihar

168. Small bitter gourd, Kaprol which is native to Vietnam and founnd in Tainwan, Hong Kong, China and India.
     (a) *Momordica charantia*   (b) *Momordica dioica*
     (c) *Momordica balsamina*   (d) *Momordica cochinchinensis*

169. Which type of Naphthalene acetic acid (powder form) is used to promote rooting in stem cuttings of Kakrol?
     (a) Planofix   (b) Seradix B, No.2
     (c) Sephadix   (e) Ceresan

170. *Balm or lemon balm* (biliiotam) the leaves of which are used as a spice and flavurant is obtained from.
     (a) *Mentha arvensis*, Labiatae
     (b) *Lavendula vera*, Labiatae
     (c) *Rosmarinus officinalis*, Labiatae
     (d) *Melissa officinalis*, Labiatae

171. Which part of *Laurus nobilis*, sweet bay Laurance is used as a spice
     (a) Leaves   (b) Stem
     (c) Roots   (d) Seeds

172. Which part of *Chervil Baz-atrila, Antihriscus cerefolium*, Umbelliferace is used as a spice
     (a) Leaves   (b) Flowers
     (c) Roots   (d) Seeds

173. Which part of *hyssop, Zufah-yob's* (*Hyssopus officinalis*, Labiatae) is used as a spice (condiment)
     (a) Leaves   (b) Flowering tops
     (c) Seeds   (d) Roots

174. What is the content of iodine in one kg of *Hyssop* plants?
     (a) 14 mg   (b) Zero
     (c) 4 mg   (d) 40mg

175. *Kokam butter* an idible fat used to ulcerations and fissures of lips, hands etc; as an adulterant of ghee, is obtained from kernels of
     (a) *Garcinia indica*, Guttiferace
     (b) *Garcimia mangostana*, Guttiferae
     (c) *Madhuca indica*, Sapotaceae
     (d) *Minusops elengi*, Sapotaceae

176. *Cassava (Manihot esculenta* Euphorbiaceae) is a
    (a) Starch crop of temperate regions
    (b) Sugar crop of sub-tropical regions
    (c) Fibre crop of tropical regions.
    (d) Starch crop of tropical regions.

177. The Bitterness in Bitter *Cassava* is due to high content of
    (a) Starch
    (b) Hydrocyanic acid
    (b) Oxalic acid
    (d) Sugar

178. The alkaloid linamarin is present in which part of *Cassava* (tapioca) plant?
    (a) Starch grains
    (b) Outer periderm of tuber
    (c) Cortex of tuber
    (d) Pitch of tuber

179. Which of the following plants contain *insecticides*?
    (a) Roots of *Tephrosia vogelii*, Papilionaceae
    (b) *Tuber of Veratrum album*, Liliaceae
    (c) Seeds of *Croton tiglium*, Euphorbiacea
    (d) Roots of *Heliopsis longipes* Asteraceae

180. Prickly pear (*Opuntia* sp.) in Australia was brought almost completely under control after the introduction of the predator.
    (a) *Chrysolina hyperici*, Beetle
    (b) *Drosophila melanogastor*, fruit fly
    (c) *Meloidogyne*, nematode
    (d) *Cactoblastis cactorum*, Bug

181. The chromosome number of *betel-vine* (*Piper betle*) is
    (a) Same as that betel palm (*Areca catechu*)
    (b) Greater than that of betel palm
    (c) Less than that of betel palm
    (d) One chromosome less than betel palm

182. Supply of *chaohar seski*; (from *Artemisia maritima*) useful in expulsion of intestinal worms and effective in intermittant remittent fevers is obtained from
    (a) Lahaul Valley in Himachal Pradesh
    (b) Astor and Gilgit in Kashmir
    (c) Kishtwar in Kashmir
    (d) All these

183. Devdaru, *Cedrus deodara*, Pinaceae is indicated in Ayurvedic medicine in
    (a) Ascites, cough, diarrhoea and dysentery
    (b) Dropsy gravel in Kidney and bladder
    (c) Headache and heart palpitation, inflammation leprosy
    (d) Paralyses, pulmonary troubles, urinary diseases, ulcers and skin diseases.

184. Oil much used for preserving *leather bags* used for floating in water.
    (a) Castor oil   (b) Til Oil
    (c) Mustard oil   (d) Cedrus wood oil

185. *Kelon-ka-tel* the best repellant to insects and fleas is obtained from
    (a) Castor Seed   (b) Til Seed
    (c) Flax seed   (d) Cedrus wood

186. Which of the following are used to make *screens* to ward off heat-wave in summer.
    (a) *Tribulus terrestris*, gothru, Zygophyllaceae
    (b) *Peganum, harmala*, Harmal, Zygophyllaceae
    (c) *Cynodon dactylon*, Poaceae
    (d) *Fagonia cretica* Dhuansa, Zygophyllaceae

187. Amino acids found in the leaves of bhringaraj, *Eclipta alba*, Asteraceae
    (a) Leucine, Isoleucine
    (b) Valine, Phenylalanine
    (c) Methionine, glycine, glutamine
    (d) Glutamic acid, cysterine

188. Which of the following are medicinal users of bhringarag, *Eclipta alba* leaves?
    (a) Ear and eye troubles, headache
    (b) Hepatic and spleen enlargement, liver cirrhosis; live protector against toxic drug and alchohol.
    (c) Skin diseases, toothache and wind trouble
    (d) All these

189. Tea leaves quickly dried after gathering, so that their colour and other characters are retained.
    (a) Black tea   (b) Green Tea

(c) Brick tea   (d) Tea dust

190. Tea leaves drived sometime after being gathered, and after
     they have undergone a king of fermentation, by which their
     original green colour is changed.
     (a) Green tea   (b) Black tea
     (c) CTC tea   (c) Brick tea

191. Which part of *Santalum album*, sandal wood, chandan yields
     essential oil, containing santanol?
     (a) Sapwood   (b) Heartwood
     (c) Bark   (d) Seeds

192. The drug *chaohar-seski* comes from which part of *Artemisia
     maritima*, Asteraceae.
     (a) Leaves   (b) Roots
     (c) Flowers   (d) Half open buds with a
                                          few leaves

193. The scales used by perfume master; where different scents
     are used to create masterpieces is called
     (a) Notes   (b) Series
     (c) Mixtures   (d) Fixatives

194. *Ambrette* perfume is obtained from the seeds of
     (a) *Abelmoschus esculentus*   (b) *Abelmoschus moschatus*
     (c) *Hibiscus micranthus*   (d) *Abutilon indicum*

195. *Everlasting* perfume is obtained from
     (a) *Dipteryx odorata*   (b) *Vanilla planifolia*
     (c) *Resedo'odorata*   (d) *Angelica archangelica*

196. *Dil of ivy*, is obtained from which part of *Hedera helix*?
     (a) Leaves   (b) Roots
     (c) Flowers   (d) Seeds

197. *Candillia wax* is obtained from
     (a) *Euphorbia antisyphilitica* (b) *Euphorbia tirucalli*
     (c) *Copernicia cerifera*   (d) *Cocos nucifera*

198. Flower of cabbage represents the sentiment of
     (a) Fame   (b) Cheerfulnews
     (c) Profit   (d) Love

199. Botanical name and family of lockat (lukat); sweet fruits which are sold in the market during the hot months March-April.
    (a) *Pyrus pyrifolia*, Rosaceae
    (b) *Eriobotrya japonica* Rosaceae
    (c) *Prunus persica* Rosaceae
    (d) *Prunus domestica* Rosaceae

200. Botanical and family of *sinhare*, an aquatic herb; fruits are edible, eaten raw or cooked; sold in markets in September-December.
    (a) *Trapa bispinosa*, Trapaceae
    (b) *Typha angustata*, Typhaceae
    (c) *Typhonium trilobatum*, Araceae
    (d) *Amorphophallus campanulatus*, Araceae

201. *Emblica officinalis (amla)* tree flowers from
    (a) March-May   (b) June-September
    (c) October - December   (d) January -February

202. *Charas* consists of which part of *Cannabis sativa*, (bhang, Indian bhang/Cannabinaceae)?
    (a) Dried leaves and flowers
    (b) Dried roots
    (c) Dried flowering tops of female plants (free from leaves)
    (d) A resinous substance which appears on the stems and inflorescence of female plant

203. The dried flowering tops of female plants (agglutinated and should be free from leaves) of *Cannabis sativa*, is called
    (a) Bhang   (b) Charas
    (c) Ganja   (d) All these

204. The drug *bharangi* (active against brochial asthama/sold in the markets of Delhi and surroundings is obtained from
    (a) Bark of *Gardenia latifolia*
    (b) Roots of *Clerodendrum serratum*
    (c) Bank of *Gardenia turgida*
    (d) All these

205. Accumulation of pottassium nitrate in the soil is indicated by the presence of which of the following plants?
    (a) *Tribulus terrestris*, Zygophyllaceae

(b) *Peganum harmala* Zygophyllaceae
(c) *Chenopodium album*, Chenopodiaceae
(d) *Fagonia cretica* Zygophyllaceae

206. Cauliflory (The flowers are borne inflorescence and also on the main trunk and braches) is seen in which of the following fruit plants?
(a) *Averrhoa carambola*, Kamrakh
(b) *Citrus limettoides*, mith of Lahore
(c) *Brassica oleracea* var *botrytis* cawliflower
(d) *Brassica oleracea* var *capitata*, cabbage

207 Which of the following plnats yield *detergenti*
(a) Fruits of hingota, *Balanites roxburghic*
(b) Fruits of ritha, *Acacia concinna*
(c) Leaves of latter *Albizia amara*
(d) Fruits of ritha *Sapindus trifoliatus*

208. Timbers suited for aircraft work
(a) Chikunda Kala *Albizzia odoratissima*; *Artocarpus hirsuta*, aini, anjili; *Betula alnoides*, bhuja patra, Indian birch; *Canarium euphyllum* dhup
(b) Safed siris, *Albizzia*, *procera*; kathal, *Artocarpus heterophyllus*, *Betula utilis*, Indian paper birch; *Canarium strictum*, Kala dammar
(c) Lallei *Albizzia amara*; chaplash, *Artocarpus chaplasha*, *Bischofia javanica*, Paniala; *Cananga odoratum*, *Cananga*
(d) *Chukrasia tabularis*, chikrassy; *Dalbergia latifolia*, Bombay black wood, *Michelia champaca* Champa; *Pterocarpus indicus*, Padank

209. Dill (*Anethum graveolens*, Apiaceae) is cultivated in
(a) India (b) Greece
(c) Indonesia (d) Malaysia

210.Fennel (*Foeniculum vulgare*, Apiaceae) is cultivaed in
(a) India (b) France
(c) Japan (d) Turkey

211. Celery seed (*Apium graveolens*) is cultivated in
(a) India (b) France
(c) Japan (d) Turkey

212. *Anise* seed (*Pimpinella turkeyandrum*, Apiaceae) is cultivated in
    (a) Turkey, Spain, Syria
    (b) India Sri Lanka, Malaysia
    (c) Haiti, Jamaica, Peru
    (d) Greece, Mexico, Italy

213. Liquorice (sweet wood) is obtained from which part of *Glycyrrhiza glabra*, Leguminoseae
    (a) Roots   (b) Rhizome
    (c) Stem   (b) Fruits

214. Which one of the following spices is an *orchid*
    (a) Ginger (*Zingiber officinale*)
    (b) Spearment (*Mentha spicata*)
    (c) Mace (*Myristica fragrans*)
    (d) Vanillin, (*Vanilla planifolia*)

215. Which one of the following spice belongs to the family Myrtaceae
    (a) Parsley (*Petroselinium crispum*)
    (b) Cumin (*Cuminum cyminum*)
    (c) Cinnamon (*Cinnamomum zeylanicum*)
    (d) Cloves (*Syzygium aromaticum*)

216. Marjoram (*Origanum majorana*), Oregano (*Origanum vulgare*) belongs to
    (a) Apiaceae   (b) Lamiaceae
    (b) Lauraceae   (d) Zingiberaceae

217. Economic use of *Sitalpati* (*Chimogyne dichotoma*, Marantaceae) is used
    (a) For stem pith ash is used as washing powder
    (b) Stem is used for making mats
    (c) Stem pith is used for making paper
    (d) Threads

218. *Sitalpati* is cultivated in
    (a) Andhra Pradesh and Tamil Nadu
    (b) West Bengal and Assam
    (c) Karnataka and Maharashtra
    (d) Rajasthan and Kashmir

219. Economic uses of anise (fruits of *Pimpinella anisum,* Umbellifereae) are
    (a) Perfuming dental preparations and mouth-washes
    (b) Flavouring foods-curries, pastry candy, bread, biscuits, beverages Liquors
    (c) A carminative which relieves flatulence
    (d) Mild expectorant; ingredient of cough syrups and lozenges

220. An important source of fruit and oil for western people for over 5,000 years
    (a) Coconut (*Cocos nucifera*)   (b) Dates (*Phoenix dactylifera*)
    (c) Olives (*Olea europaea*)   (d) Pineapple (*Ananas comosus*)

221. Which one of the following are tropical nuts?
    (a) Hazelnut, Walnut   (b) Chestnuts, Pecans
    (c) Filberts, Almonds   (d) Macadamianut, Brazil nut

222. All spice (*Pimenta dioica,* Lauraceae) is cultivated in
    (a) Spain, France, Portugal
    (b) United states, France Yugoslavia
    (c) Brazil, Srilanka Malaysia
    (d) Macadamianut, Brazil Nut

223. Saffron (*Crocus satius,* Iridaceae) is cultivated in
    (a) United States, France, Yugoslavia
    (b) Spain and Portugal
    (c) Netherlands, Poland, Denmark
    (d) Jamaica, Guatemala, Honduras, Mexico

224. Which of the following grasses stabilise shifting sandunes?
    (a) *Acacia tortilis, Calophospernum mipane*
    (b) *Cenchrus ciliaris, Lasiurus indicus*
    (c) *Dichrostachys rutans, Zizyphus nummularia*
    (d) *Prosopis juliflora, Calligonum polygonoides*

225. A drought resistant oil seed crop?
    (a) Safflower   (b) Groundnut
    (c) Dil palm   (d) Sunflower

226. *Carthamin dye* is obtained from
    (a) Safflower   (b) Sunflower

(c) Soybean   (d) Sesame

227. What is the area of salt affected soils in India?
    (a) 7 million hectares   (b) 5m hectares
    (c) 2.5 million hectares   (d) 3m hectares

228. What are the main characteristics of alkali soils?
    (a) High soil pH, often exceeding 10
    (b) Excessive amount of exchangeable and soluble sodium
    (c) Presence of calcium carboate modules, often occuring at about 1m depth
    (d) Deficiency of organic matter and available calcium nitrogen and Zinc

229. Which of the following are used to reclaim alkali soil?
    (a) Add gypsum   (b) Add urea
    (c) Add rock phosphate   (d) Add ammonia

230. Which one of the following are important to cultivated rice or wheat in a reclaimed alkali soil?
    (a) Add Zinc to the Soil
    (b) Apply more nitrogen than the normal recommended dose
    (c) Add calcium carbonate to the soil
    (d) Add ground rock phosphate to the soil

231. Which of the following are *green manure crops*?
    (a) Wheat or barley
    (b) Pearl millet or nigher
    (c) Bersem, or shaftal
    (d) Groundnut or castor

232. Ground rock phosphate (powdered) is suitable for improving
    (a) Water logged soil   (b) Acid Soils
    (c) Alkali soils   (d) Salt affected soils

233. What is the area (in million hectares) / of alkali on sodic soils in India
    (a) 1.5   (b) 4.5
    (c) 2.5   (d) 25

234. Sodic soils have high pH upto 10.7 which is due to
    (a) Excess Calcium   (b) Excess rockphosphat
    (c) Excess gypsum   (d) Excess sodium

235. Pyrite (iron sulphide Fe S) can to used to improve
     (a) Alkali soils   (b) Waterlogged soils
     (c) Acidic soils   (d) Rock phosphate soils

236. Which of the following are used in the drink *Coca-Cola*
     (a) Coca Leaves   (b) Kola seeds
     (c) Both coca leaves and (d) Coffee seeds
         Kola seeds

237. Which starch is used in the manufacutre of *vodka*, a Russian
     alcoholic drink?
     (a) Barley   (b) Rye
     (c) Potato   (d) Sugarcane

238. Which alcoholic drink is prepared from rice in Japan
     (a) Sake   (b) Vodka
     (b) Beer   (d) Whisky

239. Which alcoholic drink is flavoured with *pine resin?*
     (a) Absinthe   (b) Vermouths
     (c) Retsina   (d) Gin

240. *Gin* is flavoured with
     (a) Caraway seed   (b) Angelica root
     (c) Hops inflorescence   (d) Junior berries

241. *Brandy* is prepared from
     (a) Grapes   (b) Cereals
     (c) Apples and plums   (d) Sap

242. An alchoholic drink prepared from the leaf sap of *Agave sp.*
     (a) Calvados   (b) Slivovitz
     (c) Mezcal   (d) Tequila

243. *Gin* and *whisky* are prepared from
     (a) Grapes   (b) Fruits
     (c) Mezcal   (d) Cereals

244. *Vodka* of Russia Poland, Finland is flavoured with
     (a) Caraway (seed)   (b) Aniseed (anise)
     (c) Lime   (d) Coriander

245. *Steroidal drugs* (oral contraceptive pills, sex hormones,
     anabolics) are present in
     (a) *Dioscorea floribunda*   (b) *Dioscorea deltoides*

(c) *Dioscorea composita*   (d) All these

246. *Inulin* is present in the tubers of
(a) Cassava   (b) Yams
(c) Jerusalem artichoke   (d) Yam bean

247. Leguminous crop (pulse crops) which gives both pods (gain) and edible tubers
(a) Yam beean (*Pachyrrhizus*)
(b) Rice bean (*Vigna umbellata*)
(c) Winged beam (*Psophocarpus*)
(d) Bambara groundnut(*Vigna subterranea*)

248. Which of the following pulses contain toxic substances?
(a) Kidney Bean   (b) Black bean
(c) Soya Bean   (d) Broad bean

249. Consumption of Khesari dal cuses the disease
(a) Favism   (b) Human lathyrism
(c) Hemolytic aneemia   (d) Vitamin E deficiency

250. The alkaloid *theobromine*, which is a heart stimulant and diuretic, is present in
(a) Coca   (b) Cola
(c) Cacao   (d) Chat

251. Dried powdered roots of which plant are used to flavour or adulterate coffee?
(a) Angelica root   (b) Coriander root
(c) Chicory root   (d) Mentha root

252. A beverage plant with no caffeine
(a) Chicory   (b) Tea
(c) Chat   (d) Coffee

253. Why is it difficult to collect bamboo seed?
(a) A population of jungle mice grows too rapidly when bamboos flower and fruit.
(b) Flowering of bamboo takes place after a certain number of years of vegetative growth.
(c) Bamboos do not form seed.
(d) After the following the clump usually dies.

254. Caffeine is present in
    (a) *Annona cherimolia,* Cherimoyer
    (b) *Annona squamosa,* Sharifa
    (c) *Annona reticulata,* bullocks heart
    (d) *Annona muricata,* Sour sop

255. Main producer of carob *(Ceratonia siliqua,* Caesalpiniaceae), fruit pulp of which is used like tamarind.
    (a) Egypt   (b) Nigeria
    (c) Somalia   (d) Cyprus

256. *Locust gum* (a polymer extracted from the endosperm of seeds) is obtained from
    (a) *Bauhinia*   (b) Tamarind
    (c) *Parkinsonia*   (d) Carob

257. Coffee like beverage is prepared from the seeds of
    (a) Carob   (b) Tamarind
    (c) Gulmohar   (d) Kachnar

258. Which of the following spices are grown in India?
    (a) Dill, Fennel   (b) All spice, Caraway
    (c) Chervil, Parsley   (d) Rosemary, Thyme

259. Cassava *(Manihot esculenta)* is a
    (a) Starch crop   (b) Sugar crop
    (c) Timber tree   (d) Shade tree

260. Edible starch is obtained from
    (a) *Dioscorea bulbifera*   (b) *Dioscorea deltiodes*
    (c) *Dioscorea esculenta*   (d) *Dioscorea composita*

261. Which of the following is a host for lac insects?
    (a) Kusum   (b) Sal
    (c) Karanja   (d) Neem

262. Which of the following oil is used against headache, rheumatism and for skin diseases.
    (a) Kusum   (b) Sal
    (c) Karanja   (d) Neem

263. *Kusum oil* emits poisonous fumes at high temperature due to the presence of
    (a) Saponins   (b) Sulphur compounds

(c) Cyanogenic compounds (d) None of these

264. Which of the following is already being used in Japan, Switzerland, the U.K. and Italy, as a partial substitute for *Cocoa butter?*
     (a) Neem Fat   (b) Sal Fat
     (c) Karanja fat   (d) Kusum fat

265. Which of the following contain oil
     (a) Ambadi (mesta)   (b) Tobacco seed
     (c) Jute seed   (d) Watermelon seed

266. What is the toxic phenolic compound present in underfined cotton seed oil?
     (a) Nicotine   (b) Phenol
     (c) Theobromine   (d) Gossypol

267. Which of the following oil remain in a solid state at room termperature and can substitute cocoa butter
     (a) Sal (*Shorea robusta*)
     (b) Drumstic (*Moringa pterygosperma*)
     (c) Candlenut (*Aleurites molucana*)
     (d) Brazil nut (*Bertholletia Sp*)

268. *Safflower* is a major oil seed crop Carea of 5.15 lakh hectares) in which state of India?
     (a) Andhra Pradesh   (b) Karnataka
     (c) Maharashtra   (d) Madhya Pradesh

269. Suitably processed seed fat of which plant can be used in *confectionery* and in chocolate making
     (a) Neem, *Azadirachta indica*
     (b) Karanja, *Pongamia pinnata*
     (c) Kusum *Schleichtera oleosa*
     (d) Mahua, *Madhuca indica*

270. *Mahua cake* (left after the extraction of oil) is unfit for use as cattle feed or fertilizer. Why?
     (a) The cake is poor in nitrogen
     (b) The cake contains a toxin saponin
     (c) The cake is not palatable to cattle
     (d) The cake is a pesticide

271. Neem seed extract can be used as a
    (a) Pesticide   (b) Funguide
    (c) Rodenticide   (d) Nematicide

272. Neem Oil from the seeds of *Azadirachta Indica* is used in the Manufacture of
    (a) Edible Oil manufacture of
    (b) High quality toilet soaps manufacture of
    (c) Hydrogenated fats
    (d) Manufacture of perfumes

273. *Karanja oil* is used in
    (a) Leather tanning   (b) Lubrication
    (c) Soap making   (d) Medicinal preparations

274. *Fermentation*, drying and roasting are the processing of cocoa beans. Which microorganism helps in the following Fermentation?

$$\text{Pure Sugar} \xrightarrow{\text{(bacteria)}} \text{ethanol} \xrightarrow{\text{(bacteria)}} \text{Acetic Acid} \longrightarrow CO_2 + H_2O$$

$$\text{Pure Sugar} \xrightarrow[\text{(bacteria)}]{\text{Lactic}} \text{Lactic acid} + \text{Acetic Acid}$$

    (a) Acetic bacteria   (b) Lactic bacteria
    (c) Methanogenic bacteria   (d) Yeast

275. *Sphenoclea zeylanica* Kacharanga a weed of rice fields is useful as
    (a) Manuriae fertilizer   (b) Prevents lodging of rice
    (c) Supplies potash   (d) Helps in pollination

276. Niger (*Guizotia abyssinica*) is in an
    (a) Cereal crop   (b) Oilseed crop
    (c) Fibre crop   (d) Pulse crop

277. Little millet is
    (a) *Panicum miliaceum*   (b) *Echinochloa frementacea*
    (c) *Panium miliare*   (d) *Paspalum scrobiculatum*

278. A fodder plant suitable for cultivation in desert of western Rajasthan
    (a) *Sesbania*   (b) *Leucaena*
    (c) *Atriplex*   (d) *Lucerna*

279. Pearl millet ergotism, ragi millet poisoning, Kodo millet poisoning pearl millet polyuria these diseases in man are caused by
    (a) Bacteria
    (b) Algae
    (c) Fungi
    (d) Viruses

280. Aflatoxin isolated from *Aspergillus flavus* infected groundnut cake contains fractions B1, B2,G1,G2,M1,M2 etc. Which fraction is hepatotoxin (causes liver damage in dairy cattle poultry)
    (a) G2
    (b) B2
    (c) G1
    (d) B1

281. Out of the above fractions of aflatoxin, which is carcinogenic
    (a) G1
    (b) M2
    (c) B2
    (d) M1

282. Which oil is used by watchners as a lubricant for fine machinery
    (a) Kusum Oil
    (b) Karanja Oil
    (c) Karadi oil
    (d) Ben Oil

283. *Ben Oil* is obtained from
    (a) Sprouting broccoli
    (b) Brussel's sprouts
    (c) Seeds of sal (*Shorea robusta*)
    (d) Sees of drum stic (*Moringa oleifera*)

284. A multipurpose vegetable whose *root bark* destrous tumours and ulcers; stem bark and flowers cures dry tumours, cough and asthma
    (a) Drumstic
    (b) Chinese cabbage
    (c) Cluster beans
    (d) Snake gourd

285. *Winged bean, Xanthosoma coleus, Pachyrrhizus (Yam - bean)* are
    (a) Tuber crops •
    (b) Pulse crops
    (c) Millets
    (d) Dye yielding crops

286. 80 per cent of production of sweet potato in India, is from
    (a) Kerala and Tamil Nadu
    (b) Maharashtra and Gujarat
    (c) Aandhra Pradesh and Karnataka
    (d) Bihar and Eastern U.P.

287. Central Tuber Crops Research Institute is located at
    (a) Hyderabad   (b) Bangalore
    (c) Trivandrum   (d) Nagpur

288. *Cassava* is grown on a large scale in
    (a) Himachal Pradesh   (b) Kerala
    (c) Orissa   (d) Madhya Pradesh

289. In Indian Soils in general, application of which micronutrient increased the yield of wheat, mustard and chickpea
    (a) Zn   (b) Cu
    (c) Mn   (d) Fe

290. *Falsa*, Sweetish fruits are obtained from
    (a) Dhaman, *Grewia tiliaefolia*
    (b) Potia tree, *Thespesia populnea*
    (c) Khirni, *Manilkara hexandra*
    (d) Backain, *Melia azedarach*

291. *Khakan* oil in commerce usedin soap making obtained from
    (a) *Kydia calycina*, pula   (b) *Pterocarpus marsupium* Bija
    (c) *Salvadora persica* Pilu (d) *Salvadora olioides*, Pilu

292. Indian *gum Kino* (used in dyeing, tanning and printing) is obtained from
    (a) *Cyamopsis tetragonoloba* Guar
    (b) *Sterculia urens*, Karaya
    (c) *Astragalus gemmifer*
    (d) *Petrocarpus marsupium*, Bija

293. *Lasora* fruits (Sweet edible fruits; can be pickled) are obtained from
    (a) *Zizyphus jujuba*, Rhamnaceae
    (b) *Zizyphus nummularia*, Rhamnaceae
    (c) *Capparis aphylla*, Capparidaceae
    (d) *Cordia dichotoma*, Boraginaceae

294. Which none of the following is a very fast growing tree?
    (a) Teak (*Tectona*)   (b) White teak (gumhar)
    (c) Sal (*Shorea*)   (d) Shisham (*Dalbergia Sp*)

295. *Ground nut oil* is a
    (a) Drying oil   (b) Semi-drying Oil
    (c) **Vegetable fat**   (d) Non-drying Oil

296. *Vegetable wax* is obtained from
    (a) Fruits of bayberry, *Myrica pensylvanica*, Myricaeae
    (b) Succulent stems of, *Euphorbia antisyphilitica*, Euphorbiaceae
    (c) Leaves of *Copernicia cerifera*, Arecaceae
    (d) Seeds and stems of *Simmondsia chinensis*, Simmondsiaceae

297. *White Pepper* is obtained from
    (a) *Piper longum* (Long pepper)
    (b) *Piper nigrum* (Black pepper)
    (c) *Capsicum annum* (red pepper simla mirch)
    (d) *Capsicum frutescens* (red pepper, chillies)

298. Fruits of *belleric myrobalan (Terminalia bellerica,* Combretaceae) are used in
    (a) Flavouring foods   (b) Dyeing
    (c) Cheese making   (d) Tanning

299. *Jamun* Trees (*Syzygium cuminii* = *Eugenia jambolana*) are crooked and stunted in the Mahabaleshwar hills at 1500 mm altitude, Why?
    (a) Due to decrease in Temperature
    (b) Due to decrease in rainful
    (c) Due to decrease in relative humidity
    (d) Due to decrease in atmoshperic pressure

300. A fruit which is very rich in Vitamin C
    (a) Chebulic myrobalan   (b) Belleric myrobalan
    (c) Emblic my robalan   (d) Jamun

301. Indian almong (*deshi badam*) is
    (a) *Terminalia arjina*   (b) *Terminalia alata*
    (c) *Terminalia chebula*   (d) *Terminalia catappa*

302. Seed oil which remains solid at room temperature like kokam oil or cocoa butter and after processing can substitute cocoa butter in the chocolate industry
    (a) Sal   (b) Neem
    (c) Peepal   (d) Shisham

303. Flowers and seeds of which are rich in oil
    (a) Gumhar / White teak   (b) Mahua
    (c) Rosewood   (d) Shisham

304. The drug *Ananase - 100* contains bromelain, a proteolytic enzyme from pine applie, used to
    (a) Reducedema, ease pain, and accelerate tissure repair
    (b) Relieve cramps and spasms of the stomach.
    (c) Absorb irrit auts and provide relief.
    (d) Cure simple diarrhoea and colicky cramps

305. Which one of the following plant product is used as a histological stain?
    (a) Sfranin   (b) Indigocarmine
    (c) Cotton blue   (d) methylene blue

306. Tincture of benzoin spray is an example of a plant product used as a
    (a) Topical protectorant   (b) Bulk laxative
    (c) Antimalarial drug   (d) Topical anesthetic

307. Pain reliever *Anacin* (Standard dose) contains how many milligrams of caffeine?
    (a) 132   (b) 65
    (c) 64   (d) 32

308. A 5-oz. cup of instant coffee contains how many milligrams of caffeine?
    (a) 146   (b) 53
    (c) 110   (d) 2

309. What is the content of theobromine in dried leaves of tea?
    (a) 2.5 per cent   (b) 1.7 per cent
    (c) 3.0 per cent   (d) Zero

310. What is the content of polyphenols in dried leaves of tea?
    (a) 25 per cent   (b) 2.5 per cent
    (c) 1.7 per cent   (d) Zero

311. Which drugs from plants are used as *pain killers* in modern medicine?
    (a) Cocaine hydrochloride   (b) Camphor spirits
    (c) Tylenol with codeire   (d) Morphine sulphate

312. *Psyllium* used as laxative in medicine is obtained from
    (a) Banana leaves   (b) Karaya gum
    (c) Plantain seed husks   (d) Benzoin

313. *Cafergot* tablets which contain ergotamine tartarate (obtained from the fungus ergot) and facceine is used to treat
    (a) To stabilize heart rhythms   (b) Menstrual cramps
    (c) Migraine head headaches   (d) Diorrhea

314. Ephedrine sulphate from *Ephedra* is used as
    (a) Bronchodilator   (b) Laxative
    (c) Analgesic   (d) Anestetic

315. The drug *Lanaxin* contains digoin, a floxglove cardiac glycoside that helps to
    (a) Induce vomiting after poison ingestion
    (b) Skeletal muscle relaxation in surgery
    (c) Cure diarrhea, gastritis, colitis and nausea
    (d) Stabilize heart rhythms

316. The drug *RID* used to kill head and body lice, is obtained from
    (a) Pyrethrins   (b) Ipeacac
    (c) Pine apple   (d) Neem

317. Which of the following is a major raw material for commercial production of *steroidal drugs*, including contracetptive steroids.
    (a) Diosgenin   (b) Testosterone
    (c) Cortisone   (d) Progesterine

318. *Diosgenin* is a
    (a) Steroidal sapogenin   (b) Flasonoid
    (c) Cyclopentanoid lactone   (d) Terpenoid

319. Ovaries of 50,000 cattle could give how many grams of the *Sex hormone* progestirone.
    (a) 5100 g   (b) 500g
    (c) 250g   (d) 50g

320. Ox-bile contains the *sex hormone*
    (a) Testosterone   (b) Trogesterone
    (c) Diosgenin   (d) Cortisone

321. *Diosgenin* is extracted from which part of the jam vines *Dioscorea floribunda*, D- *composita* etc.
    (a) Leaves   (b) Flowers
    (c) Tubers   (d) Aerial stems

322. *The trade name* of a drug that includes *Rauwolfia* alkaloids that are effective in treating high blood pressure and emotional conditions
    (a) Syllact
    (b) Cofergot
    (c) Serpasil
    (d) Ananase

323. *Mayapple* yieds which compound that prevents cell proliferation in tumorous growth
    (a) Podophyllin
    (b) Empirin
    (c) Metamucil
    (d) Parapectolin

324. *Green almonds* are sold in the market as green ruts. These are obtained from
    (a) *Prunus avium*
    (b) *Prunus armeniaca*
    (c) *Prunus cerasus*
    (c) *Prunus dulcis*

325. Sex *hormone/s* which cause pollen sterility in crop plants
    (a) Norethisterone
    (b) Allylestrenol
    (b) Ethinylestradid
    (d) Levonorgestrel

326. *Contraceptive steroids* for making oral contraceptive pill, obtained from the plant *Dioscorea floribunda* are
    (a) Norethisterone
    (b) Lynestrenol
    (b) Estrogen
    (d) Progesterone

327. *Sex hormones* obtained from *Dioscorea floribunda, D. deltoidea, D. composita* are
    (a) Testosterone, Estrone, Progesterone
    (b) Cortisone, Predenisone Dexa methasone
    (c) Hydrocortisone, Prednisolone
    (d) Betamethasone.

328. *Steroidal drugs* (wonder drugs) are used in modern medicine for curing
    (a) Rheumatoid arthritis, Asthama
    (b) Inflammatory conditions, rhinitis ulcers, coloitis,
    (c) Hormonal deficiency resulting in sexual inefficiency and gynaecological disorders.
    (d) Muscular dystrophy and pituitary dwarfism

329. Kendall and Hench in 1948 discovered the treatment of rheumatoid arthritis by
    (a) Testosterone
    (b) Estrone
    (c) Cortisone
    (d) Progesterone

330. *Malay apple* (Syzygium malaccensis, Myrtaceae) is cultivated on a large scale in

    (a) Indonesia   (b) India
    (b) Malaya   (d) Burma

331. Which part of *Clove bean* (michi) are used as vegetables?
    (a) Leaves   (b) Flower buds
    (c) Roots   (d) Fruits

332. Which variety of potato is used for making popular *potato chips*?
    (a) Kufri Moti   (b) Kufri Khasi Garo
    (c) Kufri Jyoti   (d) Kufri Chandramukhi

333. In *grapes*, poor quality - sour taste, thicker skin and less pulp tissue is due to the deficiency of
    (a) Calcium, nitrogen carbohydrate
    (b) Magnesium, sulphur, calcium
    (c) Copper Zinc, Molybdeniem
    (d) Manganese, boron potassium

334. In grapes, berry drop is due to the deficiency of
    (a) Magnesium Zinc   (b) Calcium, potassium
    (c) Molybolenum, Sulphur (d) Boron, copper

335. An important fruit of Bihar
    (a) Litchi   (b) Apple
    (c) Custard apple   (d) Banana

336. Mountain spinach, an edible leafy vegetable is
    (a) *Atriplex hortensis*   (b) *Spinacia oleracea*
    (c) *Beta vulgaris*   (d) *Beta vulgaris* var
                                   bengalensis

337. Oriental pickling melon is
    (a) *Cucumis melo var conomon*
    (b) *Cucumis melo var agretis*
    (c) *Cucumis melo var momordica*
    (d) *Cucumis melo var utilissimus*

338. Unroasted, dried coffee contains how much per cent of polyphenols?
    (a) Zero   (b) 1.5 per cent
    (c) 4.5 per cent   (d) 3.6 per cent

339. *Kola* fresh seeds and guarana dried fruit contains how much per cent of theobromine and polyphenols?
    (a) Zero
    (b) 4.5 per cent
    (c) 1.5 per cent
    (d) 3.5 per cent

340. *Cocoa* fresh cotyledons contain how much per cent of thebromine?
    (a) Zero
    (b) 3.6
    (c) 2.4
    (d) 5.2

341. The beverage *mate* is obtained from which part of the plant *Ilex paraguariensis*, Aquifoliaceae
    (a) Leaves
    (b) Fruits
    (c) Seeds
    (d) Roots

342. *Mate* is a popular beverage in
    (a) Argentina
    (b) Uruguay
    (c) Southeastern Brazil
    (d) Paraguay

343. *Woad*, a source of blue dye is obtained from
    (a) *Lawsonia, inermis*, Lytheraceae
    (b) *Carthamus, tinctorius*, Asteraceae
    (c) *Rubia tinctoria*, Rubiaceae
    (d) *Isatis tinctoria*, Brassiacaceae

344. Gin and Vodka differ from whiskey in that
    (a) They contain very low percentage of alcohol
    (b) They contain very high percentqge of alcohol
    (c) They lack flavouring agents
    (d) They have lavouring agents

345. *Areca husk* is a good source of
    (a) Xylose
    (b) Furfuraldehyde
    (c) Starch
    (d) Sugar

346. The residue of *areca husk* (after extraction of xylose), when mixed with Zince chloride and heated to 800°C for 2 hours, gives
    (a) Furfural
    (b) Activated carbon
    (c) Charcoal
    (d) Hemicellulose

347. Which of the following impround varieties of *groundnut* are most suited for growing in Haryana state?
    (a) MH-1,MH-2
    (b) BP-1,BP-2

(c) M-145, TMV-8   (d) TG-1, TG-3

348 Which of the following improved varietieds of *sesamum* are most suited for growing in Orissa state?
(a) Mrug-1, Purba -1, Madhuri
(b) Kanak, Kalika, Vienayak
(c) JT-7, Pratap Gauri
(d) TC-25, N-32, T-13

349. A technique for rapid and non-destructive determination of oil in oil seeds
(a) Pulsed Nuclear Magnetic Resonance
(b) Solvent extraction method
(c) Rotary Mills
(d) Hydraulic presses

350. Which of the following are paddy field blue-gree algee
(a) *Wollea*   (b) *Aphanotheca*
(c) *Gloetrichia*   (d) *Plectonema*

351. *Which of the following are the alkaloids of acrecanut?*
(a) Arecoline, arecolidine, arecaidnine
(b) Guvacine   (c) Isoguvacine
(d) Guvacolidine

352. The anthelmintic propertis of (effective against tapeworms and round worms) *arecanut* are due to
(a) Guvacine   (b) Guvacolidine
(c) Isoguvacine   (d) Arecoline

353. What is the percentage of fat in *arecanut?*
(a) Zero   (b) 1 - 2
(c) 14-15   (d) 5-10

354. What is the percentage of tannius (polyphenols) in tender *arecanuts?*
(a) 38 - 47   (b) 6-10
(c) 16-22   (d) 22-30

355. The non-arecoline fraction of *arecanut* can be used in opthalmology
(a) As a miotic against for constricting the pupils in the eye.
(b) For curing night blindness

(c) For curing tumours in eye

(d) For stopping the falling of eye lashes.

356. *Arecanut* extract inhibits the growth of

   (a) *E. coli*   (b) *Salmonella typhi*

   (c) *Streptococcus aurens*   (d) *All these bacteria*

357. Which of the following can be chemically pulped by digest
     ing with chemicals at 170°C for 9 hours; this pulp is suitabl
     for making brown wrapping paper?

   (a) Arecanuts   (b) Arecanut husk

   (c) Areca roots   (d) Areca leaves

358. Which of the following is *palak* nutritious green leafy veg-
     etable in some pars of India.

   (a) *Chenopodium album*

   (b) *Beta vulgarius* var *cicla*

   (c) *Beta vulgarius* var *benghalensis*

   (d) *Beta vulgaris*

359. What is the botanical name of *Spnach (palak)*, a nutritious
     green leafy vegetables?

   (a) *Spinacea oleracea*   (b) *Chenopodium album*

   (c) *Beta vulgaris* var *benghalensis* (d) *Beta vulgaris*

360. *Pine-apple* is propagated vegetatively using

   (a) Suckers and slips   (b) Crowns and butts

   (c) Seeds   (d) Rhizome

361. The essential oil of coriander, mint basil, thyme, parsley
     which give flavour and aroma due to

   (a) Copper compounds   (b) Magnesium compounds

   (c) Sulphur compunds   (c) Zinc compounds

362. The economic uses of *Curry leaf tree (Murraya Koenigii,
     Rutaceae)* are

   (a) Leaves are used in cookery for flavouring food stuffs.

   (b) Leaves root and bark are tonic, stomachic and carmina-
       tive;

   (c) Root is used in piles; alley heat of human body;thirst;
       imflammation and itching; to relieve pain associatedwith
       Kidney

   (d) Leaves check vomiting; used in the treatment of dysentry
       and diarrhoea

363. *Fortified wines* are
    (a) Fermented wines to which distilled spirits are added.
    (b) Fermented wines to which a little extra sugar is added and tightly capped
    (c) Fermented wines to which CO_2 is added and tightly capped.
    (d) Fermented wines to which yeast is added.

364. What is the chromosome number (2n) of coconut?
    (a) 38   (b) 34
    (c) 40   (d) 32

365. 2-or 6 - rowed inflorescence is a character of
    (a) Barley   (b) Oat
    (c) Rye   (d) Buckwheat

366. Which of the following cereals has grain capable of germinating at 1°C above freezing and naturing when temperatures are as low as 12°C (55°F)
    (a) Rice   (b) Wheat
    (c) Oat   (d) Rye

367. *Dry breads* are made with half wheat and half rye flour, and not with rye flour along, why?
    (a) Rye seed protein is useless for making light bread
    (b) Wheat seed protein is useless for making light bread
    (c) Wheat and rye proteins are usefull for making heavy bread
    (d) None of these

368. Which Nitrogen fixing blue-green alga is always found in the cavities on the dorsal leaves of the aquatic ferm, *Azolla*?
    (a) *Wollea*   (b) *Aphanotheca*
    (c) *Anabaena*   (d) *Plectonema*

369. Oyster mushroom, dhingri, a kind of edible mushroom is
    (a) *Agaricus campestris*   (b) *Agaricus bisporus*
    (b) *Morchella* sp.   (d) *Pleurotus sajorcaju*

370. Which of the following Chemical present germination of paddy grain is submerged rice plants (due to heavy downpour cyclones etc)
    (a) Sodium chloride   (b) Bleaching powder
    (c) Maleic hydrazide   (d) Potassium chromate

371. Which of the following orchids are rare species?
    (a) *Venda coerulea* (blue vanda)
    (b) *Paphiopedilum venustun* (lady's slipper orchid)
    (c) *Cymbidium elegans*
    (d) *Anoectochilus roxburghi* (jewel orchid)

372. Australian grape varieties resistant to pests and diseases; suitable for growing in hot, humid, coastal areas?
    (a) Campbell Early   (b) Catawba
    (c) Lady Patricia   (d) Carolina Blackose

373. In Netherlands, which of the following *orchids* are cultivated in test tubes?
    (a) *Cymbidium*   (b) *Gerbera*
    (c) *Anthurium*   (d) All these

374. In India, arid zone occupies which per cent of the area
    (a) 12   (b) 24
    (c) 2   (d) 34

375. In arid zones of India, with facility of water hearvesting which fruits can be grown
    (a) Jugube   (b) Pomegranate
    (c) Guava   (d) Custard apple

376. In arid zones, with supplementary irrigation which fruit crops can be cultivated?
    (a) Mango   (b) Banana
    (c) Amla   (d) Sour Line

377. In arid Zones, undwer assured irrigation, which fruit crops can be cultivated
    (a) Grapes, papaya   (b) Data palm
    (c) Mulberrt   (d) Phalsa, sweet orange

378. Butter cup banyan (Makhan katori) is
    (a) *Ficus bengalensis* (b) *Ficus*
    (c) *Ejcus*   (d) *Ficus Krishna*

379. *Vanda coerulea* (blue orchid) is native to the hills of
    (a) Nilgiris   (b) Mahabaleshwar
    (c) Khasi   (d) Aravalli

380. Main constituent of *cassia oil* is
    (a) Cinnamic aldehyde   (b) Eugenol

(c) Pinene   (d) Cineol

381. *Saigon Cassia* is
   (a) *Cinnamomum zeylanicum* true cinnamon
   (b) *Cinnamomium cassia*, cassia
   (c) *Cinnamomum burmannii*, Pedang cinnamon
   (d) *Cinnamomum laureiril* Royal cinnamon

382. About 80 per cent of the total imports of *Cassia* into the United Staes belongs to
   (a) *Cinnamomum burmannii*, Batavia cassia
   (b) *Cinnamomum laureirii*, Saigon cassia
   (c) *Cinnamomum cassia*, Cassia China
   (d) *Cinnamomum zeylanicum*, true Cinnamon

383. Russia and Germany prefer which of the following for *flavouring chocolates*?
   (a) Cassia buds   (b) Cinnamon buds
   (c) Indian cassia bark   (d) Cassia bark

384. The leaves of which of the following are used mainly as a spice
   (a) *Cinnamomum tamala*
   (b) *Cinnamomum zeylaniucum*
   (c) *Cinnamomum aromaticum (C. cassia)*
   (d) *Cinnamomum iners*

385. *Khoker cloves* are
   (a) Cloves which have undergone fermentation due to improper drying
   (b) Clove fruits produced as a result of the fertilisation of the opened flower bud
   (c) Cloves without the ball shaped unopened flower bud at the top
   (d) All these

386. *Decaldehyde* used in perfumery is obtained by treating *coriander* seed oil with
   (a) Water   (b) Ethyl alcohol
   (c) Benzene   (d) Bisulphite

387. The oleoresin obtained from coriander seeds is used to flavour
   (a) Beverages   (b) Sweets

(c) Pickles   (d) All these

388. Superesin obtained from *Coriander* seed is
    (a) Soluble coriander   (b) Volatile oil
    (c) Decaldehyde   (d) Residue after distilling oil

389. *Black cumin* is obtained from the dried seed-like fruits of
    (a) *Cuminum cyminum*, Umbelliferae
    (b) *Nigella sativa*, Umbelliferae
    (c) *Anethum sowa*, Umbelliferae
    (d) *Foeniculum vulgare*, Umbelliferae

390. *Anethum graveolens* is
    (a) Indian dill   (b) European dill
    (c) Fennel   (d) Fenugreek

391. The fiterous sponge of which fruit has attained international
    usage as filters for naval engines, bath sponges, table mats,
    bathroom mats, slipper soles, insulation for sound-proof
    boards, abrasives for cards glassware and Kitchen-ware.
    (a) *Luffa cylindrica*, ghia tori
    (b) *Luffa acutangula* Kali tori
    (c) *Momordica charantia*, Karela
    (d) *Trichosanthes anguina* Chichinda

392. Botanical name of fenugreek (meth)
    (a) *Trigonella foenum-graecum*   (b) *Cyamopsis tetragonoloba*
    (c) *Fleminga strobilifera*   (d) *Uraria prunellaefolia*

393. Important *aromatic* barks which are in commercial use are
    (a) True Cinnamon, *Cinnamomum zeylanicum*
    (b) Jangli darchini, Kareeva, *Cinnamomum iners*
    (c) Tejpat, *Cinmamomum tamala*
    (d) Ram tejpat, *Cinnamomum obtusifolium*

394. *Cassia* used as a spice is
    (a) Jangli-darchini, *Cinnamomum iners*
    (b) Tejpat, *Cinnamomum tamala*
    (c) Ram tejpat, *Cinnamomum detusifolium*
    (d) True cinnamon, *Cinnamomum zeylanicum*

395. *Indian Cassia* Legnea (Indian cassia bark) is
    (a) True cinnamon *Cinnamomum zeylanicum*
    (b) Jangli darchini, *Cinnamomum iners*

    (c) Tejpat, *Cinnamomum tamala*

    (d) Ram Tejpat, *Cinnamomum zeylanicum*

396. *Cassia china* is

    (a) True cinnamon, *Cinnamomum zeylanicum*

    (b) Cassia, *Cinnamomum Cassia*

    (c) Tejepat, *Cinnamomum tamala*

    (d) Raw tepat, *Cinnamomum obtusifolium*

397. *Cassia lignea* of commercce is

    (a) True cinnamon, *Cinnamomum zeylanicum*

    (b) Cassia, *Cinnamomum cassia*

    (c) Tejpat, *Cinnamomum tamala*

    (d) Ram tejpat, *Cinnamomum obtusifolium*

398. *Kala Nagkesar (Cassia* buds) of commerce are the unripe fruits of

    (a) *Cinnamomum zeylanicum*   (b) *Cinnamomum tamala*

    (c) *Cinnamomum obtusifolium* (d) *Cinnamomum cassia*

399. True **Jumiper berries** are adulterated with berries of

    (a) *Juniper communis* var *nana*

    (b) *Juniper oxyeedrums*

    (c) *Pinus wallichiana*

    (d) *Abies pindrow*

400. *Welsh onion* is

    (a) *Allium porrum*   (b) *Allium fistulosum*

    (c) *Allium sativum*   (d) *Allium cepa*

401. *Mace* is the dried reticulated aril of

    (a) *Ricinus*   (b) *Pithecellobium*

    (c) *Polygala*   (d) *Myristica*

402. When the peach or apricot - like nutmeg fruit bursts open, the mace is seen as an attractive bright scarlet cage closely enveloping or clothing the hard, thin, black shining shell of the seed called

    (a) Mace   (b) Blade of mace

    (c) Strophile   (d) Nutmeg

403. In India, *nutmeg* is grown in

    (a) Araku valley(Andhra Pradesh)

    (b) Wynad (Kerala)

(c) Nilgiris, Burliar, Coimbatore, Salem, Ramandhapuram Tirunelveli, ' Kanyakumar, Madurai(Tamil Nadu)

(d) Assam

404. Pure *mace* is adultered with
   (a) *Myristica fragrans*
   (b) *Myristica malabaricum*
   (c) Both of these
   (d) None of these

405. *Mace* volatile oil is used in
   (a) Flavouring liquor
   (b) Flavouring tobacco
   (c) Flavouring dental creams
   (d) All these

406. Economic uses of *galangal* (Kulanjan) are
   (a) In rheumatism and catarrhal affection, specially in bronchial catarrh.
   (b) Respiratory troubles, especially of children
   (c) Carminative and stomachic
   (d) Depressant of the cardio - vascular system

407. What are the economic uses of *garlic / lassar (Allium satium,* Liliaceae)?
   (a) As a condiment in mayonnaise producs, salad dressings, tomato products and in several meat preparations.
   (b) Contains an antibiotic allicin which shows antibacterial action.
   (c) Raw garlic can be used in the garlic paste garlic salt, garlic vinegar, garlic cheese croutins, garlicked potato chips, garlic bread, garlicked meat tit-bits and garlickede bacon.
   (d) Garlic juice is used against ailments of stomech, as a rubefacient in skin diseases, and as ear drops in ear-ache. Leaves are used in the treatment of asthma.

408. *Horse-radish*, a highly prixed condiment specially with oysters, cold meats, boilded or roasted beef, shring, cocktail etc. is the fleshy root of
   (a) *Raphanus sativus,* Cruciferae
   (b) *Daucus carota,* Umbelliferae
   (c) *Rorippa indica,* Cruciferae
   (d) *Cochlearia armoracia,* Cruciferae

409. Crushed *horse-radish* has an inhibitory effect an the growth of micro -- organisms, this effect is being attributed to
   (a) Ascorbic acid
   (b) Sulphur

(c) Glucoside   (d) Allyl isothiocynate

410. The diried leaves and flowering tops of *savory* are derived from
(a) *Satureia hortensis*, Labiatae
(b) *Ocimum kilimandscharicum*, Labiatae
(c) *Rosmarinus officinalis*, Labiatae
(d) *Salvia spendens*, Labiatae

411. *Savory*, an erect rubescent annual herb is found in
(a) Kashmir India   (b) Southern France
(b) Germany, Spain   (d) England, Canada, US

412. Users of *Savory* as a condiment
(a) Flavouring of soups and sources
(b) Egg, salad dished, poultry dressing
(c) Pork sausage and any other sausage
(d) Fish, Stews, Salads, sauces

413. *Vamillin* is obtained from
(a) *Cuminum* sp.   (b) *Vanilla planifolia*
(c) *Coriandrum*   (d) *Anethum graveolens*

414. R. Hacines (1856), J. Stenhouse (1855) have shown that crystals obtained from oil of *ajowan* (*Trachyspermum*) *ammi sys. Carum copticum*), sold in Indian markets under the name of *ajouwan ka phul* or *sat ajowan* is identical to
(a) Vanillin   (b) Eugenol
(c) Decaldehyde   (d) Thymol

415. The chief constituent of *oil of thyme* (*Thymus vulgaris*, banajwain, Labiatae)
(a) Vanillin   (b) Eugenol
(c) Decaldehyde   (d) Thymol

416. *Galangal* a spice, is produced from which part of *Alpinia galanga*, Zingiberaceae
(a) Fruits   (b) Leaves
(c) Stem   (d) Rhizome

417. Which of the following *greater Cardamoms*
(a) *Amomum aromaticum*, Bengal cardamom
(b) *Amomum kepulaga*, Round cardamom
(c) *Amomum subulatum* Nepal cardamom

(d) *Elettaria cardamomum,* Malabar cardamom

418. Which of the following is called *Grains of Paradise*
    (a) *Amomum aromaticum*　　(b) *Amomum kepulaga*
    (c) *Aframomum melegueta*　　(d) *Amomum subulatum*

419. Lesser cardamom, *small cardamom, chhota Elaichi* are
    (a) *Elettaria cardamomum* var minuscula
    (b) *Elettaria cardamomum* var major
    (c) *Aframomum angustifolium*
    (d) *Amomum aromaticum*

420. What are the economic uses of *celery seed (Apium graveolens,* Umbelliferae)
    (a) Celery seeds are used as a spice; leaves and stalks are used as Salads in soups
    (b) Used against asthma and liver diseases
    (c) Seeds are used as nervine sedative and tonic; remedy fro rheumatism
    (d) Celery seed oil is used in flavouring food producs, clery salts, celery tonics and culinary sauces.

421. Botanical name of *celeriac,* used as a spice
    (a) *Apium graveolens*
    (b) *Apium graveolens var rapaccum*
    (c) *Anthriscus cerefotium*
    (d) *Anethum graveolens*

422. Which glucoside is present in *Caper buds* which on hydrolysis, gives rhamnox, dextrose and Quercetin.
    (a) Saponin　　　　　　(b) Pectiv acid
    (b) Oleic acid　　　　　(d) Rutin

423. On acid hydrolysis rutin gives rhamnose, dextrose and Quercatin, On hydrolysis by the enzyme rutinease, rutin yields
    (a) Quercetin　　　　　(b) Rutinose
    (c) Rhammnose　　　　(d) Dextrose

424. Rutinose, a sugar, on acid hydrolysis gives
    (a) Quercetin　　　　　(b) Rhamnose
    (c) Dextrose　　　　　(d) All these

425. Capsicum or Chillies which are restricted to South and Central America
    (a) *Capsicum frutescans,* Solanaceae
    (b) *Capsicum pendulum,* Solanceae
    (c) *Capsicum pubescans,* Solanceae
    (d) *Capsicum annum,* Solanaceae

426. Botanical name of caraway, shia jira
    (a) *Carum bulbocastanum* Umbelliferae
    (b) *Apium graveloens,* Umbelliferae
    (c) *Cuminum cyminum* Umbellifrae
    (d) *Carum carvi,* Umbelifreae

427. Which of the following is Madagascar Cardamom
    (a) *Aframomum angustifolium,* Zingiberaceae
    (b) *Aframomum hannburyi,* Zingiberaceae
    (c) *Aframomum Korarima,* Zingiberaceae
    (d) *Aframomum melegueta,* Zingiberaceae

428. A variety of *sweet basil* (*Ocimum basilicum,* Labiatae) - lettuce leaf basil is
    (a) *Ocimum basilicum* var *purfurascens*
    (b) *Ocimum basilicum* ver *thyrsiflorum*
    (c) *Ocimum basilicum* var *differne*
    (d) *Ocimum basilicum* var *album*

429. Which type of *sweet basil* oil is produced in Europe and is highly prized for its fine odours
    (a) Oil which contains methyl chavicol as the principal constituent and linalool, but no camphor.
    (b) Oil which contains methyl chavicol and camphor, no limalool
    (c) Oil which contains mehtyl charicol, linalool and a substantial amount of methyl cinnamate but no camphor
    (d) Oil which contains eugenol as the main constituent

430. *Sweet basil seeds* when steeped in water, liberate a mucilage; the mucilage yields on hydrolysis
    (a) Glucose　　　　　　　　(b) Uronic aicd
    (c) Xylose　　　　　　　　 (d) Rhamnose

431. *Laurel leaves* or bay leaves, the dried leaves of *Laurus nobilis*, Lauraceae are cultivated in
    (a) Greece amd Spain   (b) Asia Minor
    (c) Central America   (d) Portugal

432. *Caper buds* (Kalera) *Capparis spinosa*, Capparidaceae are very usefull in curing
    (a) Scurvy (Vitamin C deficiency)
    (b) Beri Beri (Vitamin B, deficiency)
    (c) Rickets (Vitamin D feficiency)
    (d) Night blindness (Vitamin deficiency)

433. Economic uses of *caper buds* are
    (a) Flavouring fish and meat sources
    (b) As a garnish in cold roasts and salads
    (c) Caper source with boiled mutton is a favourite in Wes:-ern countries
    (d) Flavouring pickles and relishes

434. What are the economic uses of *Lemon balm* (*Melissa officinális*, Labiatae) used as a spice
    (a) Fresh or powdered leaves are used in fish dishes, stuffing or as a substitute for lemons
    (b) The fruit is considered a brain tonic and is usefull in hypochondriac conditions.
    (c) Leaves and stems are useful is brain, liver and heart diseases and also in bites of venomous insects.
    (d) Lemon balm is said to possess stomachic, anti-tubercular and anti- pyretic properties; it is used to strengthen the gems and to remove bad taste from the mouth

435. *Amchur* is obtained from
    (a) Unripe fruits of *Mangifera indica*
    (b) Fruits of *Tamarindus indica*
    (c) Leaves of *Hibiscus cannabinus*
    (d) Ripe fruits of *Mangifera indica*

436. Which of the following spice contains the steroidal substances diosgenin which is used as a starting material in the sysnthesis of sex hormones, and oral contraceptives
    (a) Asafoetida *Ferula asafoetida*
    (b) Carrot, *Daucus carota*

    (c) Fenugreek, *Trigonella foenum-graecum*
    (d) Bishops weed *Carum copticum*

437. What are the medicinal user of *Fenugreek* (methi) seed
    (a) Used in colic flatulence, dysentery, diarrhoea
    (b) Used in dyspepsia with loss of appetite, chronic cough, dropsy
    (c) Used to cure enlargement of liver and spleen, rickets, goat and diabetes
    (d) Infusion is given to small pox patients as a cooling drink; used in sweets served to ladies during the post-natal period.

438. The mushroom *Amanita muscaria* got its name fly-agaric or *fly mushroom* due to its property of
    (a) The spores fly in the air
    (b) Causing hallucinations of flying in air
    (c) Attracting and killing insects
    (d) Forming food for flies

439. *Rauwolfia, Vinca, Cannabis* and *Arisaema* lead the long list of plants of Himalayas known to and used in medicine today. What is the economic importance of *Arisaema* (Araceae)
    (a) Root is used as snake- bite antidote
    (b) The plant accumulates crystals of calcium oxalate
    (c) The plant causes irritant dermatitis
    (d) All these

440. Which of the following plant families are found at extemely high elevations in the Himalayas?
    (a) Papaveraceae   (b) Magnoliaceae
    (c) Caryophyllaceae   (d) Euphorbiaceae

440a. A plant (the only plant) Apiaceae (Umbelliferae) which contains alkaloids?
    (a) *Conium maculatum*   (b) *Coriandrum sativum*
    (c) *Carum copticum*   (d) *Angelica archangelica*

441. One of the famous plant poisons used by ancient Greeks. The famous Greek philosopher Socrates was made to drink the poison from this plant.
    (a) *Conium maculatum*   (b) *Amanita muscaria*
    (c) *Nerium indicum*   (d) *Thevetia peruvina*

442. Plants used to maintain *low blood sugars* in humans
    (a) Tea made from *Daucus carota*, carrot
    (b) Tea made from *Catharanthus roseus*, Periwinkle
    (c) Tea made from *Eurya theoides*
    (d) Tea made from *Camelia sinensis*

443. Plants used for the control of *diabetes* insulin subsitutes.
    (a) Tecomine and Tecostanine from *Tecoma stans*
    (b) Immature bean pods, olive leaves, potatoes,
    (c) Wheat, celery, blckberry leaves, sugarbeet
    (d) Leaves and roots of banana

444. Plants showing hypoglycemic activity (*control of diabetes*)
    (a) *Lycopodium clavatum; Taxus cuspidata*
    (b) Cashew plant, *Rhus typhina*, celery, coriander, carrot, snake root, ginseng, *Oplopanax horridum*
    (c) Coconut lettuce, sunflower, Jerusalem artichoke dandelion, papaya, peyote, sweet potato, Karela
    (d) Methi, pea, onion, garlic banana, allspice, olive, oats, barley, corn tobacco, ginger

445. Plants used for the control of *gout* (acute attacks of gouty arthritis)
    (a) Gibberellin from *Fusarium moniliforme*
    (b) Fruits of Quince *Cydinia oblonga*
    (c) Colchicine from *Colchicum autumnale*
    (d) Fruits of sweet *cherry, Prunus avium*

446. *Sugar substitutes* from plants
    (a) Monellin (*Dioscore phyllum cumminisii* berries); Perillartine (essential oil of *Perilla frutescens*);
    (b) Steviaside (leaves of *Stevia rebaudiana*); Glycyrrhizin (roots of *Glycyrrhiza glabra*, licorice)
    (c) Naringin (fruit of *Citus paradise*) Neohesperidin
    (d) Osladin (rhizome of *Polypodium vulgare*); Diastereoisomeric diterpene acids from Pinus resin

447. Taste -modifying *sugar substitutes* (persistent sweet taste for few hours)
    (a) Miraculin (berry of *Synsepalum ducificum*)
    (b) Gymnemic acids (leaves of *Gymnema sylvestre*)
    (c) Chlorogenic acid, Cynarin (*Cumara scolymus*)

(d) Maltol (larch bark, pine needles, roasted malt, *chicory*)

448. Plant which cures liver diseases
   (a) Dandelon roots (*Taraxacum officinale*)
   (b) Fruit of *Emblica officinalis* amla
   (c) *Rumex verticillatus*, roots, of *Solidago nemoralis* to cure jandice.
   (d) *Salix lucida* (removing bile from the stomach) *Zanthoxylum clava- herculis* (for obstructions) of the liver

449. Ancient European cures for liver complaints
   (a) *Hepatica nobilis* Ranunculaceae
   (b) Thallus of liver worts
   (c) Mosses
   (d) Pteridiophytes

450. A widely used species in the *toothpastes* of the Asian subcontinent
   (a) Neem, *Azadirachta indica*
   (b) Tipal, *Ficus religiosa*
   (c) Bargad, *Ficus benghalensis*
   (d) Harra, *Terminacia chebula*

451. In Jamaica, a *mouthwash* known as *Chew-Dent* is the plant extract of
   (a) *Acacia Senegal*, Mimosaceae
   (b) *Salvadora persica*, Loganiaceae
   (c) *Peltophorum Sp*, Fabaceae
   (d) *Gouania lupulioedes*, Rhamnaceae

452. Which alga is used commercially as an abrasive *dentifrice* (Sodium algenate thickener)
   (a) *Mactrocysits*, Brow alga   (b) *Fucus Sp.*, Brown alga
   (c) *Laminaria Sp*, Brown alga (d) *Ecklenia Sp.*, Brown alga

453. Botanical name of *toothbrush tree*, powdered stem of which is used as an abrasive dentifrice in central America
   (a) *Conmiphora myrrha*, Burseraceae
   (b) *Lannea grandis*, Anacardiaceae
   (c) *Krameria triandra*, Krameriaceae
   (d) *Gouania lupuloides*, Rhamnaceae

454. Chrwing sponges for *cleaning teeth*, are a popular means of tooth cleaning in Ghana. Such material in market places in Ghana are
    (a) *Acacia pennata*
    (b) *Hibiscus rostellatus*
    (c) *Lasianthera africana*
    (d) *Terminalia glaucescens*

455. Alkaloids present in *hembock (onum)* maculatum
    (a) Coniine, methylconincie
    (b) Coniceine
    (c) Conhydrine
    (d) All these

456. Main symptoms of *hemlock(Conium maculatum)* poisoning
    (a) Dilation of pupils, rapid respiration
    (b) Difficulty in movement, particularly of the hind limb
    (c) The pulse at first low, becomes rapid and therady, temperature lowered
    (d) Death due to respiratory failure

457. The first alkaloid to be produced synthetically in the laboratory
    (a) Coniine
    (b) Coniceine
    (c) Conhydrine
    (d) Methylconiine

458. It causes those devouring it to be able to foresee and predict things; such as weather on the following day the enemy will make an attack upon them or weather will continue favourable; or to discern who has stolen from them some utensils or any thing else ". Eating of which of the following plant grants powers about future?
    (a) Ergot grain of *Claviceps purpurea*, Ergot fungus
    (b) *Lophophora williamisii* peyote cactus, miscal button
    (c) *Psilocybe mexicana*, Sacred mushroom
    (d) *Amanita caesaria*, a mushroom

459. The cleaned mushroom, after boiling passed through burning incense were apporitioned in pairs to those attending the ceremony visions of palace gardens covered with precious stones came into view soon after. also, visions of unreality of many sorts came to the participants ". After eating which mushroom?
    (a) *Amanita phalloides*
    (b) *Amanita muscaria*
    (c) *Agaricus bisporus*
    (d) *Agaricus campestris*

460. *Brochoditators* relax the smooth muscles of the bronchioles, the small bronchial tubes in the lungs that lead to the air cells, thereby diminishing generalised peripheral airway obstruction. A plant used as bronchodilator and to relieve bronchial asthma.

(a) *Ephedra gerardiana*, Ephedraceae

(b) *Euphorbia hirta*, Euphorbiaceae

(c) *Glycyrrhiza glabra*, Fabaceae

(d) *Monarda fistulosa*, Lamiaceae

461. Root infusion of which plant is specific for curing, *asthma and bronchitis* in India.

(a) *Euphorbia hirta*, Euphorbiaceae

(b) *Glycyrrhiza glabra*, Fabaceae

(c) *Tylophora Indica*, Asclepiadaceae

(d) *Verbascum thapsus*, Scrophulariaceae

462. Plants trusted in domestic and aboriginal medicine as efficacious for *respiratory diseases*

(a) *Ephedra, Tylophora indica; Saussurea lappa, Costus (Asteraceae)*

(b) *Lobelia inflata*, Indian tobacco((Campanula); *Euphorbia hirta; Glycyrrhiza glabra* licorice; *Verbascum thapsus*

(c) *Monarda fistulosa*, Laamiaceae; *Datura stramonium; Alpinia galagal*, greater galangal, Zingiberaceae

(d) All these

463. Plants used now in China for treating chronic bronchitis

(a) *Rhododendron anthopogonoides*, Ericaceae

(b) *Ardisia japonica, A. hortorum*, Myrsinaceae

(c) *Bergina sibirica*, Saxifragaceae

(d) All these

464. Normally *teeth* are extracted surgically, but according to folklore they may be *removed* readily if treated with

(a) The powder from dried roots of the celandine poppy, *Chelidonium majus*

(b) Latex from *Chlorophora tinctoria*, Moraceae

(c) Latex from *Hura crepitans, Euphorbiaceae*

(d) Seed oil from *Ximenia americana*, Olacaceae; bark of *Acacia pennata* soaked in palm wine

465. A type of chewing gum called *bubble gum* is obtained from
    (a) *Mimusops balata*   (b) *Achras zapota*
    (c) *Sideroxylon glabrescens*   (d) *Ficus platyphylla*

466. *Spanish herbal cigarettes* for curing coughs, colds, bronchitis, asthma, and pulmonary complaints, are made from leaves of
    (a) *Nicotiana tabacum*, Solanaceae
    (b) *Datura Stramonium*, Solanaceae
    (c) *Hyoscyamus niger*, Solanaceae
    (d) *Atropa belladonna*, Solanaceae

467. Leaves of *Datura* species used in cigarettes smoking for relief of *asthma*, in various parts of the tropics.
    (a) *Datura stramonium*   (b) *Datura metel*
    (c) *Datura fastuosa*   (d) All these

468. A 19th century home remedy in Europe, included dried flowers or roots of which plant, used as cigarettes for *asthmatics*.
    (a) *Camellia sinensis*, Theaceae
    (b) *Tylophora indica*, Asclephiadaceae
    (c) *Saussurea lappa*, Asteraceae
    (d) *Verbascum thapsus*, mullein, Scrophulariaceae

469. Plants used as *expectorants* (used orally to stimulate patients to cough, thereby relieving their chest congestion
    (a) Ipecac syrup (*Cephealis ipeacuanca*) mixed with cherry or raspberry syrups
    (b) Cined from Eucalyptus, wormseed and rosemary
    (c) Pinene from pine, juniper and other gymnosperms; creosote from *Fagus ferruginea*
    (d) Terpin hydrate synthesized from geraniol (*Pelargonium odoratissimum*)

470. Planted used as *mucolytic agents* (used to clear the chest of sputum
    (a) Leaves of *Adhatoda vasica*, Acanthaceae
    (b) Leaves of *Eriodictyon californicum* yerba santa Hydrophyllaceae
    (c) *Apocynum androsaemifolium*, *A. cannabinum* Apocynaceae
    (d) *Acalypha indica*, *Euphorbia corollata*, *E. Ipecacuanta* (ipecapurge), Euphorbiaceae

471. The sacred mushrooms of Mexico, called *"Flesh of the Gods"* which contain many hallucinogenic alkaloids
     (a) *Conocybe*   (b) *Panaeolus*
     (b) *Psilocybe*   (c) *Stropharia*

472. Plants used as *nasal snuff*, for intoxication (South American Snuffs)
     (a) *Virola*, sp. Myristicaceae
     (b) *Justicia pectoralis* Acanthaceae
     (c) Ashed bark of *Elizabetha princeps*, Fabaceae
     (d) All these

473. *Stim-u-Dents*, a type of toothpicks recommended by periodontists are made from Stim-u-Dents are dispensed in some commercial airlines for after meal cleaning
     (a) Fruiting pedicals of *Ammi Visuaga*, Apiaceae
     (b) *Salix alba, Salix jessoensis*, Willows
     (c) *Populus* sp. polar with peppermint
     (d) Wood of balsa (*Ochroma lagopus*), flavored with peppermint and colored orange

474. Tooth-cleaning fruit
     (a) *Agelaea obliqua*   (b) *Cnestis ferruginea*
     (c) *Azadirachta indica*   (d) *Feronia limonia*

475. Which of the following are present in *international toothpastes* in commerce
     (a) Green arabic, gum Karaya, gum tragacanth
     (b) Mucilages from marine red algae (Carrageenan or Irish moss and *Grigaxtina mamillosa*), brown algae (algin from *Laminaria, Macrocystis and Nereocystis*)
     (c) Volatile oils from spemint, caraway, Cinnamon, peppermint, cloves, thymus, pimenta, anise, nutmeg, Sassafras
     (d) Volatile oils from sweet orange, bitter orange, lemon eucalyptus, wintergreen

476. Centre of origin of *wheat*
     (a) South America
     (b) North central North America
     (c) United States
     (d) Central Asia

477. Centraep of production of *groundnut*
     (a) India   (b) China
     (c) S. America   (d) Ethiopia

478. Centre of origin of *potato*?
     (a) Peru   (b) Eastern Europe
     (b) Hawaii   (d) United States

479. In recent years there has been great interest in the production of which mycotoxin from *Aspergillus flavus* which grows rapidly on moist peanut cake.
     (a) Lycomarasmin   (b) Alternaric acid
     (c) Enniatin   (d) Aflatoxin

480. *Tung Oil* used in China for waterproofing wood, paper and fabric; in the manufacuture of paints, varnishes, enamels and lacquers is obtained from which part of *Aleurites* montana, A. fordiu from which part of *Aleurites montana, A. fordii* (Euphorbiceae)
     (a) Wood   (b) Kernals of fruit
     (b) Roots   (d) Leaves

481. *Kekuna oil* used in paint and varn sh industries, for making candles; for culinary purposes; as a luminant; hair tonic; substitute of from oil is obtained
     (a) *Aleurites montana*, Euphorbiaceae
     (b) *Aleurites fordii*, Euphorbiaceae
     (c) *Euphorbia hirta* Euphorbiaceae
     (d) *Aleurites moluccana*, Euphorbiaceae

482. Place of origin ginseng, *Panax ginseng*, Araliaceae
     (a) Northeastern United States   (b) Siberia
     (c) Korea   (d) Manchuria

483. *Hallucinogenic drugs* - d-lysergic-acid amide, d-isolysergic-acid amide are present in
     (a) *Rivea corymbosa* oldiuqui, Convolvulaceae
     (b) *Ipomoea Violacea*, granni-vine, Convolvulaceae
     (c) *Methysticodendron amesianum*, culebra borrachera, Solanaceae
     (d) *Duboisia hopwoodii*, pituri, Solanaceae

484. In South America, the wood of *Quebrach* (*Schinopsis lorentzii*, Anacardiaceae) provides
     (a) Timber   (b) Dye

(c) Tannin   (d) All these

485. Wood tree (*Isatis tinctoria* Cruciferae) yields
    (a) Timber   (b) Dye
    (c) Tannin   (d) All these

486. Fill up the blank?
    ——————— acrinyl isothiocynate + dextrose + sinapin hydrogen sulphate
    (a) Erucic acid   (b) Volatile mustard oil
    (c) Sinalbin   (d) Sinigrin

487. Sinalbin is present in
    (a) White mustard   (b) Black mustard
    (c) Rocket cross   (d) Indian rape

488. Economic use of *olive oil* (*Olea eropaea*, Oleaceae)
    (a) For edible purposes, in cooking, salad oils and food preservation
    (b) Sardine fish canning
    (c) High class toilet preparations and cosmetics also in pharmaceuticals
    (d) In the textile industry, it is used in wool combing.

489. *Kheersal* a natural product, collected from the cavities of old trees, much used as a remedy in relaxed throat. It is sweetish and astringent in taste. Kheersal is obtained from the wood of
    (a) *Acacia catechu*   (b) *Acacia arabica*
    (c) *Acacia senegal*   (d) *Acacia leucophloea*

490. The leaves of which of the following *Acacia* species yield a *gree dye* with turmeric
    (a) *Acacia catechu*   (b) *Acacia farnesiana*
    (c) *Acacia leucophloea*   (c) *Acacia concinna*

491. Rod Bark or stan bark is used to *flavour spirits* prepared from sugar cane and palm juice
    (a) *Acacia leucophloea*, safed Kikar
    (b) *Acacia arabica*, babul Kikar
    (c) *Acacia senegal*, Kher
    (d) *Acacia concinna*, ritha

492. Bark can be used as a substitute for wattle bark in the *tanning* of skins
   (a) *Acacia leucophloea*, safed Kikar
   (b) *Acacia arabica*, babul
   (c) *Acacia catechu*, khair
   (d) *Acacia concinna*, ritha

493. *Gum arabic* of commerce is obtained from
   (a) *Acacia pennata*   (b) *Acacia arabica*
   (c) *Acacia leucophloea*   (d) *Acacia senegal*

494. *Cassie perfume* is distilled from the flowers of
   (a) *Acacia pennata*   (b) *Acacia concinna*
   (b) *Acacia leucophloea*   (d) *Acacia farnesiana*

495. Pods are used for *washing silk*, wollen fabrics and for cleaning tarnisned silver plates
   (a) *Acacia catechu*   (b) *Acacia senegal*
   (c) *Acacia concinna*   (d) *Acacia arabica*

496. The starchy edible seeds called *maiz del aqua* or *water corn*, in parts of South America are obtained from
   (a) *Nelumbium speciosum*, lotus
   (b) *Nymphaea stellata*, Indian blue water-lily
   (c) *Nymphaea lotus*, chota kamal
   (d) *Victoria regia*, giant water lily

497. The flower of which orchid is considered to be the lucky flower in Sri Lanka and is used as a temple offering at a Buddhist festival during May. The flowers are locally called *Wesak mala* (May flower)
   (a) *Dendrobium maccarthial* (b) *Zeuxine sulcata*
   (c) *Vanda tesellata*   (d) *Cypripedium elegans*

498. The deliciously scented *orchid fruits* are
   (a) *Dendrobium*   (b) *Corallorhiza*
   (c) *Habenaria*   (d) *Vanilla*

499. In Mauritius, tasty "*Laham tea*" is prepared from the dried leaves of which orchid
   (a) *Geodrum densiflora*   (b) *Angracum fragrans*
   (c) *Calanthe veratrifolia*   (d) *Vanilla planifolia*

500. Plant producing biggest flower (3 ft in diameter)
    (a) *Raphia raffia*   (b) *Hibiscus rosa-sinensis*
    (c) *Rafflesia arnoldi*   (d) *Puja raimondii*

501. Which of the following plant products is extensively used as
    a composite food for the *in vitro* culture of plant cells, tissues
    and organs
    (a) Coconut milk   (b) Agar agar
    (c) Potato starch   (d) Sugar

502.

    The above diagram is the chemical structure of
    (a) Pinene   (b) Taxol
    (c) Colchicine   (d) Diosgenin

503. *Chalmoogra Oil (Taraktogenos kurzii Syn-Hydnocarpus kurzii*

    Flacourtiaceae) is used in the treatment of
    (a) Pulmonary pneumonia   (b) Tuberculosis
    (c) Jaundice   (d) Leprosy

504. Fruits of *Chenopodium ambrosioides var. anthelminticum* Amer-
    ican *weed*, Chenopodiaceae is active against
    (a) Round worms   (b) Hookworms
    (c) Skin diseases   (d) Ringworm

505. Botanical name of *Sweet Chestnut*
    (a) *Castanea sativa*, Fagaceae
    (b) *Castanea denta*, Fagaceae
    (c) *Castanea Crenata*, Fagaceae
    (d) *Castanea mollissima* Fagaceae

506. *Sweet almond* is
    (a) *Prunus dulcis* var. *amara*, Rosaceae
    (b) *Prunus dulcis* var. dulcis, Rosaceae
    (c) *Prunus domestica* subsp. *institia*, Rosaceae .
    (d) *Prvnus lauroceasus*, Rosaceae

507. *Oyster nut* of East Africa
    (a) *Canarium ovatum*, Burseraceae
    (b) *Castanospermum australe*, Leguminosae
    (c) *Bertholletia excelsa*, Lecythidaceae
    (d) *Telfairia pedata*, Cucurbitaceae

508. Botanical name of *filbert*
    (a) *Corylus maxima*, Corylaceae
    (b) *Corylus avellana*, Corylaceae
    (c) *Juglans regia*, Juglandaceae
    (d) *Juglans nigra*, Juglandaceae

509. *Opium* is a narcotic obtained as a
    (a) Juice from the injured unripe capsules of *Papaver somniferum*
    (b) Resin from leaves, flowers, seeds and stems of *Cannabis sativa*
    (c) White crystalline alkaloid from *Erythroxylon coca*
    (d) All these

510. Which of the following plants is a source of *Cocaine*
    (a) *Erythroxylon coca*   (b) *Coffea arabica*
    (c) *Camellia sinensis*   (d) *Theobroma coca*

511. *Panama rubber* is obtained from
    (a) *Ficus elastica*   (b) *Castilla elastica*
    (c) *Ficus infectoria*   (d) *Ficus hispida*

512. *Assam* or *India rubber* is obtained from
    (a) *Ficus elastica*   (b) *Ficus glomerata*
    (c) *Ficus hispida*   (d) *Ficus infectoria*

513. A drug from plant which can control the growth of ovarian, breast and lung *cancer tumours*
    (a) Taxol from *Taxus*   (b) Taxol from *Taxodium*
    (c) Taxol from *Taraxacum*   (d) Taxol from *Abies*

514. What is the major discovery by medical researchers regarding *Taxol*, in 1979.
    (a) Taxol condenses chromosomes
    (b) Taxol interacts with tubulin, a protein involved in cell division
    (c) Taxol interferes in DNA replication
    (d) Taxol interferes in the formation of cell wall

515. Which of the following plants is used as *cure for almost all diseases* in China
    (a) *Panax quinquefolia*, ginseng
    (b) *Panax ginseng*, ginseng
    (c) Both of these
    (d) None of these

516. Which part of *ginseng* is used in medicine?
    (a) Leaves   (b) Seeds
    (c) Flowers   (d) Roots

517. Roots of *Heliopsis longipes, H. helianthoides, Tephrosia vogelie, Tripterygium wilfordii* are used as
    (a) Tonic   (b) For curing diseases
    (c) Dyes   (d) Insecticide

518. Herculin, Neoherculin used as minor *insecticides* are obtained from
    (a) *Ryania speciosa*, Flacourtiaceae
    (b) *Quassia amara*, Simaroubaceae
    (c) *Veratrum album*, Liliaceae
    (d) *Zanthoxylum clava herculis*, Rutaceae

519. *Oil of pepper*, obtained by the steam distillation of crushed black pepper is used in
    (a) Flavouring sausages, canned meat
    (b) Flavouring soups
    (c) Flavouring beverages
    (d) All these

520. `King of Spices' is
    (a) Red pepper   (b) All spice
    (c) Jamaican pepper   (d) Black pepper

521. Which of the following are *Soft woods*
    (a) Pine   (b) Spruce
    (c) Cedar   (d) Fir

522. *Eagle wood* or the true agar of commerce is obtained from
    (a) Wood of *Pterocarpus marsupium*
    (b) Wood of *Santalum album*
    (c) Wood of *Chloroxylon swietenia*
    (d) Wood of *Aquilaria agallocha,*

523. The wood of *Aquilaria agallocha*, agar, *agaru* becomes highly scented when it is loaded wish an oleo-resinous matter, the result of infection by
    (a) Alga   (b) Fungus
    (c) Bacterium   (d) Virus

524. *Natural paper* is obtained from the bark of
    (a) *Azadirachta indica*   (b) *Ficus benghalensis*
    (c) *Santalum album*   (d) *Aquilaria agallocha*

525. A catechu known as *Kossa*, is obtained by boiling arecanut (*Areca catechu*, Palmae) with
    (a) Water   (b) Lime
    (c) Salt   (d) Oil

526. Economic uses of a semi-drying oil obtained from the seeds of *Argemone mexicana*, bharband, Papaveraceae
    (a) It is used as a luminant, lubricant
    (b) As a preventive of white ants
    (c) In the manufacture of soap
    (d) As a substitute for linseed oil; used by painters

527. A favourite wood for musical instruments
    (a) *Artrocarpus chaplasha*   (b) *Artocarpus heterophyllus*
    (c) *Azadirachta indica*   (d) *Psidium guajava*

528. *Cultivated fig* is
    (a) *Ficus racemosa*   (b) *Ficus carica*
    (c) *Ficus benzamina*   (d) *Ficus lucescens*

529. Which part of *Papaver somniferum* plant, opium poppy contain more morphine
    (a) Stigmas   (b) Yellow dry head
    (c) Whole green head   (d) Stem

530. India imports *pellitory root*, (*Anacyclus pyrethrum*, Asteraceae) indicated in apoplexy, gingivitis, headache, lethargy cases, pain, paralytic affections, rheumatism, typhus fever and chewed as masticatory for toothache
  (a) North Africa (Algiers)   (b) Russia
  (c) Egypt   (d) Sudan

531. *Isabgol* (aswagol) indicated in chronic diarrhoea, constipation, gastro-intestinal and genito-urinal tracts troubles, rheumatism and gout (paste applied) is obtained from which part of *plantago ovata*, plantaginaceae
  (a) Leaves   (b) Stem
  (c) Fruit husk   (d) Roots

532. *Gum ghati* is obtained from
  (a) *Acacia arabica*   (b) *Acacia catechu*
  (c) *Acacia concinna*   (d) *Acacia pennata*

533. *Cutch*, a brown or yellow orange dye used for cotton, sails, silk, cordage fishing nets, canvas bags and in calico printing is obtained from which part of Khair, *Acacia catechu*
  (a) Root   (b) Bark
  (c) Leaves   (d) Heart wood

534. *Katha*, used as an antioxidant for vegetables oils, used for masticatory with *pan and supari* is obtained from which part of *Acacia catechu*
  (a) Root   (b) Bark
  (c) Leaves   (d) Heartwood

535. Members of Apiaceae (Umbelliferae) fruits or seeds of which are used for *tea*
  (a) *Anethum graveolens*, dill; *Angelica archangelica*, angelica
  (b) *Carum carvi*, caraway; *C. roxburghianum*
  (c) *Foeniculum vulgare*, fennel
  (d) All these

536. *Flowers* used as teas throughout the world
  (a) *Artabotrys uncinatus*, Annonaceae; *Borago officinalis*, Boraginaceae; *Croton crymbulosus*, Euphorbiaceae
  (b) *Tilia cordata*, linden (Tiliaceae)
  (c) *Citrus sineusis*, seville orange; *Citrus lemon* lemon
  (d) *Roupala montana*, Proteaceae; *Malva sylvestris*

537. *Barks* used as *teas* throughout the world
    (a) *Catha edulis*, chat, Celastraceae
    (b) *Cylopia subterenata*, Fabaceae
    (c) *Aniba canelilla*, Lauraceae
    (d) *Roupala montana*, Proteaceae

538. Leaves of which plant are used in South Africa as a source for commercially available *Caspa Tea*
    (a) *Cyclopia subterenata*, Fabaceae
    (b) *Catha edulis*, *chat*, Celastraceae
    (c) *Trigonella coerulea*, Fabaceae
    (d) *Rosa canina*, *Rosa pomifera*, Rosceae

539. Leaves of which plant are used in Russia for preparing *Kapporie* or *Kapor tea*
    (a) *Rhus aromatica*, Anacardiaceae
    (b) *Ceanothus americanus*, Rhamnaceae
    (c) *Listea novleoutes*, Lauraceae
    (d) *Epilobium angustifolium*, Onagraceae

540. Root used to *flavor cigarette tobacco*
    (a) Angelica   (b) Purple angelica
    (c) Coriander   (d) Chamomile

541. Dried flower heads contain a volatile oil for *flavouring cigarette tobacco*
    (a) Chamomile   (b) Nutmeg
    (c) Mace   (d) Coriander

542. *Tree tobacco*, leaves of which contains an alkaloid anabasin; Indians in western United States use these leaves for smoking
    (a) *Nicotiana tabacum*   (b) *Nicotiana glauca*
    (c) *Nicotiana trigonophylla*   (d) *Nicotiana rustica*

543. *Indian tobacco*, leaves of which are smoked by North-Indians, Americans, Chile.and in India
    (a) *Lobelia excelsa* (Campanulaceae)   (b) *Lobelia inflata*
    (c) *Lobelia tupa*   (d) All these

544. Leaves smoked for curing *tonsilities*
    (a) *Sauropus quadrangularis*, Euphorbiaceae
    (b) *Nicotiana tabacum*, Solanaceae

    (c) *Nicotiana glauca,* Solanaceae

    (d) *Nicotiana rustica,* Solanaceae

545. Widely used with betel leaves; extensively used in medicine for the treatment of asthma; sold in Japan as " *Sim-Sim* " tablets

    (a) Cutch tanin from *Acacia catechu*

    (b) Khaki obtained from *Acacia catechu*

    (c) Kheer sal from *Acacia catechu*

    (d) Kattha from *Acacia catechu*

546. Szent Gyorgyi, Hungarian scientist was awarded Nobel Prize in 1937 for isolating *vitamin C* in

    (a) Paprika, *Capsicum annuum*

    (b) Chillies, *Capsicum frutescens*

    (c) *Capsicum pendulum*

    (d) *Capsicum pubescens*

547. Cultivated species of capsicum are C.*annuum,* C.*frutescens,* C.*chinense,* C. *pendulum and* C. *pubescen* are

    (a) Southern California   (b) Spain, Hungary

    (b) Bulgaria, Yugoslavia   (d) South and Central America

548. The *Vanilla* sticks of commerce are the

    (a) cured stems   (b) Cured fruits

    (c) Cured leaves   (d) Cured roots

549. *Vanilla* is obtained from

    (a) *Vanilla fragrans,* Orchidaceae

    (b) *Vanilla planifolia,* Orchidaceae

    (c) *Vanilla pompona,* Orchidaceae

    (d) *Vanilla tabitensis,* Orchidaceae

550. During curing process, *Vanilla* pods get the flavour due to

    (a) Action of β-glucosidase on glucovanillin

    (b) Presence of alcohol

    (c) Presence of protein

    (d) Presence of resins

551. Wheat are the uses of *Vanilla* (vanillin) besides flavourant of food and perfumery

    (a) Foaming in lubricating oils can be prevented; anti-oxidant

(b) Brightener in Zinc plating baths

(c) Aid for the oxidation of linseed oil

(d) Solubilizing agent for riboflavin (Vitamin B_2)

552. The *spice* which yields four spices - bark and wood, leaf oil, berry oil, dried unripe berries used for flavouring condiments.

    (a) Pimenta   (b) Coriander

    (c) Cumin   (d) Fenugreek

553. The English `Jamaica pepper' and the German 'Nelkenpfeffer' is

    (a) Pimenta   (b) Pimento

    (c) Cumin   (d) Fenugreek

554. *Allspice* is the "four spices - in-one " and contains the flavour of

    (a) Cloves   (b) Nutmeg

    (c) Cinnamon   (d) Black pepper

555. Another name of *Allspice*

    (a) Pimenta   (b) Pimento

    (c) Cloves   (d) Nutmeg

556. Which of the following shows bactericidal, fungicial and anti-oxiandant properties

    (a) Pimenta bark   (b) Pimenta wood

    (c) Piementa leaf oil   (d) Pimenta berry oil

557. The name *allspice* is derived from the fact that

    (a) The plant yields berries, berry oil, leaf oil, bark and wood used as condiment.

    (b) The berries are used curry powders, mincemeat spice, pastey spice, poultry dressing, frankfurter, hamburger etc.

    (c) The berries contain the flavour of cloves, nutmeg, cinnamon and black pepper

    (d) The plant yields essential oils from bark and wood, leaves and berries

558. Match the following cucurbits

    (a) Snake gourd   1. *Cucumis melo var. flexuosus*

    (b) Snake melon   2. *Cucumis melo var. saccharinus*

(c) Persian melon   3. *Cucumis melo var. reticulatus*

(d) Honeydew melon   4. *Trichosanthes anguina*

559. Match the following *cucurbits:*

   (a) Pomegranate melon   1. *Cucumis metiliferus*

   (b) Oriental pickling melon   2. *Cucumis melo var. chilo*

   (c) Mango melon (orange melon) 3. *Cucumis melo var. conomon*

   (d) African horned melon   4. *Cucumis melo.*

560. Match the following *cucurbits*

   (a) Malabar melon   1. *Cucurbita ficifolia*

   (b) Winter squash   2. *Cucurbita mixta*

   (c) Missouri gourd   3. *Cucurbita foetidissima*

   (d) Hedgehog gourd   4. *Cucumis dispaccus*

561. Which one of the following is used as a bathing brush?

   (a) *Cucurpita pepo*

   (b) *Momordica charantia*

   (c) *Luffa acutangula*

   (d) *Trichosanthes anguina*

562. *Abrasive dentifrices* of natural origin, used for cleaning teeth?

   (a) Powedered root of *Acorus calamus*; powdered fruit of *Myrobalanifera,* sp. Combretaceae

   (b) Powdered bark of *Cinchona officinalis*; ashes of burned branches of *Vitis vinifera*

   (c) An infusion of the cortex of *Caesalpinia pulcherrima, Gaultheria procumbens*, winter green roots

   (d) Pulverized barks of *Alnus glutinosa* (black alder), Myrica *Pensylvanica* (bay berry) and *Quercus velutina* (black oak) to which was added one part *Asarum canadense* (American wild ginger) powdered rhizome.

   The *sugar beet* plant, *Beta vulgaris* var. *rapa.* Brassicaceae

   a) Produces seeds in the first year

   b) Produces seeds in the second year

   c) Reproduces with the help of thickened roots

   d) Never produces seeds.

564. *Swede or rutabaga, a vegetable* of recent origin grown in Europe
   (a) *Brassica napus*   (b) *Brassica napobrassica*
   (c) *Brassica raper*   (d) *Brassica vulgaris*

565. Which of the following *vegetables* belong to Liliaceae (Alliaceae)
   (a) Onion, grlic   (b) Ciboule, rakkyo, chives
   (c) Shallot, leek   (d) All these

566. Which of the following are tuber crops
   (a) Oca, ullucu or melloco
   (b) Anu, arracacha, Yam bean, maca
   (c) Sweet potato, potato, cassava, yams, aroids, arrow root
   (d) All these

567. *Fruits* of Solanaceae
   (a) Cape gooseberry, *Physalis peruviana*
   (b) Pepino, *Solanum muricatum* .
   (c) Naranjilla, *Solanum quitoense*
   (d) Tree tomato, *Cyphomandra betacea*

568. *Celtuce* is
   (a) Asparagus lettuce   (b) Only lettuce leaves
   (c) Spnach leaves   (d) Cabbage lettace or head
       lettuce

569. Match the following
   (a) *Lactua sativa var capitata*   1. Head lettuce
   (b) *Lactuca sativa var longifolia*   2. Romaine lettuce
   (c) *Lactuca sativa var crispa*   3. Curled lettuce
   (d) *Lactua sativa var asparagina*   4. Asparagus lettuce

570. The leaves are not palatable as they are coarse, and only the interiors of the young fleshy stems are consumed, after cooking?
   (a) Head lettuce
   (b) Cos lettuce (Romaine lettuce)
   (c) Curled lettuce
   (d) Asparagus lettuce (Celtuce)

571. Plants used as cure *arthritis* including rheumatism

    (a) *Aralia racemosa*, spikenard; *Chimaphila umbellata*, spotted winter green;

    (b) *Gentiana catesbaei*, blue gentian; *Hamamelis virginana*, with rhazel; *Monarda punetata*, horsemint

    (c) *Phytolacca americana*, poke; *Sanguinaria canadensis* (blood root)

    (d) All these

572. Folk remedies to treat *arthritis*

    (a) Apple cider vineager

    (b) Lugol's solution (iodine)

    (c) Honey

    (d) Parkelp (algal tablets)

573. Match the following:

(a) Cauliflower	1. *Brassica oleracea var botrytis*
(b) Cabbage	2. *Brassica oleracea var capitata*
(c) Knolkhol (Kholrabi)	3. *Brassica oleracea var gongyloides*
(d) Brussels sprouts	4. *Brassica oleracea var gemmifera*

574. Match the following:

(a) Chinese cabbage, pak-choi	1. *Brassica oleracea var. gongyloides*
(b) Chinese cabbage, pe-tsai	2. *Brassica oleracea var acephala*
(c) Kale	3. *Brassica pekinensis*
(d) Bandh Gobhi	4. *Brassica chinensis*

575. *Rheum rhaponticum*, rhubarb (Polygonaceae) is one of the most acidic of all vegetables, the juice having a pH of

    (a) 10.2   (b) 7.0

    (c) 5.8   (d) 3.2

576. Which phenomenon renders the leaves of salad (*Lactuca sativa*, Compositae) unfit for human consumption

    (a) Shortening of stem

    (b) Thickening of the fleshy step

    (c) Lactiferous leaves

    (d) Bolting

577. Botanical name of *New Zealand Spinach*
    (a) *Spinacia oleracea*, Chenopodianceae
    (b) *Tetragonia tetragoniodes*, Aizoaceae
    (c) *Lactnea sativa* (Compositae)
    (d) *Mollugo alisinoides* (Aizoaceae)

578. Match the following varieties of tomato
    (a) Cheery tomato   *Lycopersicon esculentum var cerasiforme*
    (b) Potato leaves tomato   *Lycopersicon esculentum var grandifolium*
    (c) Pear tomato   *Lycopersicon esculentum var pyriforme*
    (d) Common tomato   *Lycopersicon esculentum var commune*

579. Ancestor of all cultivated tomatoes
    (a) *Lycopersicon esculentum* var *cerasiforne*
    (b) *Lycopersicon esculentum* var *calidum*
    (c) *Lycopersicon esculentum* var *gradiflorum*
    (d) *Lycopersicon esculentum* var *pyriform*

580. Which of the following plants of *compositae* are eaten as *fodder* by the cattle
    (a) *Ageratum conyzoides*,   nilam, tombakoo, bhakumbar
    (b) Asteraceae   rissa.
    (c) *Volutarella ramosa*, rissa   rukhri, bai surai
    (d) *Pluchea lancelata rukhri*, rissa   bano, barna.

581. *Globe artichoke*, hatichuk, *Cynara scolymus* is a member of
    (a) Brassicacae   (b) Asteraceae
    (c) Capparidaceae   (d) Acanthaceae ·

582. *Lactuca sativa, salad*, grown as green vegetable for its crisp, edible, radical leaves is a member of the family.
    (a) Brassicaceae
    (b) Asteraceae
    (c) *Capparidaceae*
    (d) *Umbelliferae*

583. A plant of Compositae which gives a strong smell of *turpentine*
    (a) *Blumea obliqua*   (b) *Blumea bifoliata*
    (c) *Blumea mollis*   (d) *Blumea lacera*

584. The plant of Compositae, the roots of which possess a faintly aromatic odour
    (a) *Blainvillea latifolia*   (b) *Vigiueria helianthoides*
    (c) *Helianthus tuberosus*   (d) *Tridax procumbens*

585. Botanical name of and family of *Jerusalem artichoke hatipitch*, cultivated for its edible tubers
    (a) *Solannum tuberosum*, Solanaceae
    (b) *Daucus carota*, Umbelliferae
    (c) *Raphanus sativus*, Cruciferae
    (d) *Helianthus tuberosus*, Compositae

586. *Marmelle oil*, an essential oil is distilled from
    (a) Fruit rind of *Citrus reticulata*, Rutaceae
    (b) Fruit rind of *Citrus sinensis*, Rutaceae
    (c) Fruit rind of *Citrus lemon*, Rutaceae
    (d) Fruit rind of *Aegle marmelos*, Rutaceae

587. Which of the following are *true*?
    (a) Meseal, a strong fiery beverage is prepared from the roasted leaves of *Agave americana*
    (b) The sap that exudes on lopping the flowering stalk of *Agave americana*, *A. sisalana* is made into pulque beer.
    (c) Mexial brandy is made from the sap of the flowering stalk (by distilling) of *A. americana* and *A. sisalana*. Sugar and Vinegar are made from the sap
    (d) All these.

588. Wood of *Ailanthus excelsa, the tree of Heaven* is suitable for
    (a) Making match boxes .
    (b) Making match sticks
    (c) Making fishing floats, country boats, catamaran
    (d) Making newsprint, packing cases.

589. The aromatic resin that exudes from cuts made in the bark is used as incence and in the manufacture of *agarbattis*
    (a) *Ailanthus excelsa*, Simarubaceae
    (b) *Ailanthus triphysa*, Simarubaceae
    (c) *Ocinum Kilimindscharicum*, Labiatae
    (d) *Ocinum sanctum*, Labiatae

590. Leaves of which plant is used by market gardeners to cover immature fruits, like mangoes, plantains, custard apples, etc.

to hasten ripening to ensure development of their natural colour and to prevent them from becoming mouldy

(a) Leaves *Solanum nigrum*, Solanacea

(b) Leaves of *Annona squamosa*, Annonaceae

(c) Leaves of *Magnolia grandiflora*, Mangnoliaceae

(d) Leaves *Adhatoda vasica*, Acanthaceae

591. The stem of which plant is used for making *mukut* (marriage crowns for Hindu brides and bridgrooms, *shera* (the bridal viel of Muslims)

(a) *Aeschynomane aspera*

(b) *Ochroma lagopus*

(c) *Tectona grandis*

(d) *Sesbania sesban*

592. Charcoal prepared from this plant is in demand for making gun powder and *fire works*

(a) *Tamarindus indica*   (b) *Casuarina equisetifolia*

(c) *Acacia arabica*   (d) *Aeschynomena indica*

593. Wood is used as fuel for *firing pottery*

(a) *Tamarindus indica*   (b) *Casuarina equisetifolia*

(c) *Acacia arabica*   (d) *Aeschynomene indica*

594. The leaves and twigs provide *fodder* of excellent quality

(a) *Albizzia lebbek*, Siris

(b) *Albizzia amara*, Lallei

(c) *Albizzia odoratissima*, Kala Siris

(d) *Albizzia procera*, white siris

595. The tree supplies hooked sticks for the Himalyan rope *bridges*, the wood makes good match sticks but not match boxes

(a) *Alstonia scholaris*, rhatan, Apocynaceae

(b) *Aleurits moluccana*, Japhal akrot, Euphorbiaceae

(c) *Albizzia procera*, white siris, Leguminosae

(d) *Alnus nitida*, sharaol, Betulaceae

596. *Ditta bark* of commerce is obtained from

(a) *Alstonia scholaris*, shaitan, Apocynaceae

(b) *Aleurites moluccana*, Japhal akrot, Euphorbiaceae

(c) *Albizzia procera*, white siris, Leguminosae

(d) *Alnus nitida*, sharol, Betulaceae

160 *Question Bank*

597.˙ The oil extracted from the woody shell of the nut of *Anacardium occidentale, Kaju* Anacardiaceae is usefull in the manufacture of
  (a) Insualting varnished, type-writer rolls,
  (b) Automobile break linings, industrial flooring tiles, oil- and acid- proof cold setting cements.
  (c) Good baking enamels, finishing reagents, inks, oil cloth, paints
  (d) All these

598. *Wine, Vinegar* and pleasant beverages are prepared from
  (a) Woody shell of nut of *Anacardium occidentale*
  (b) Seed of *Anacardium occidentale*
  (c) Wood of *Anacardium occidentale*
  (d) Apple of *Anacardium occidentale*

599. Paper is made out of the waste leaf material left over after extracting the fibre of
  (a) *Ananas comosus*, pine-apple, Bromeliaceae
  (b) *Annona Squamosa*, sitaphal, Annonaceae
  (c) *Anogeissus latifolia*, dhaura, Combretaceae
  (d) *Anthocephalus indica*, Kadam, Rubiaceae.

600. *Pyrethrum* insecticidal preparations are obtained from
  (a) *Chrysanthemum cinerarifolium*, Asteraceae
  (b) *Chrysanthemum roseum*, Asteraceae
  (c) *Chrysanthemum marschalli*
  (d) All these

601. *Rotenone*, an insecticide is obtained from
  (a) *Derris elliptica, D.tripoliata, D. malaccensis, D.ferruginea*
  (b) *Lonchocarpus urucue, L. utilis*
  (c) *Tephrosia, Milletia*
  (d) *Mundulea, Sophora*

602. *Alcoholic beverages* (spirituous liquors) are obtained from
  (a) *Borassus flabellifer*, palmyra palm, Palmae
  (b) *Cocos nucifera* flower spathe
  (c) Drupes of *Grewia asiatica*, Tiliaceae
  (d) Seeds of *Punica granatum*, Punicaceae

603. Plants used for *flavouring* country *liquor* and as adjuncts in the fermentation of sugar
    (a) Root bark of *Acacia arabica*, bark of *A. leucophloea*
    (b) Leaves and root stocks of *Acorus calamus*
    (c) Leaves of *Punica granatum*
    (d) Leaves of *Cassia occidentalis*

604. The *gum* of that exudes from the bark of which of the following plant is used as a size in the manufacture of *Nepal paper*
    (a) *Albizzia procera*, Safed siris
    (b) *Albizzia odoratissima*, Kala siris
    (c) *Albizzia lebbecky* siris
    (d) *Albizzia amara*, Varacchi

605. Fungus galls of *Haplophragmium* and *insect galls* occur on the tree
    (a) *Acacia leucophloea*   (b) *Acacia catachu*
    (c) *Acacia auriculiformis*   (d) *Acacia modesta*

606. The tree is a *host for lac insects*
    (a) *Acacia leucophloea*   (b) *Acacia catechu*
    (b) *Acacia catechu*   (d) *Acacia ferruginea*

607. Leaves are eaten as *fodder* by *goats* and other animals
    (a) *Acacia leucophloea*   (b) *Acacia arabica*
    (c) *Acacia catechu*   (d) *Acacia concinna*

608. The tree is an important source of *Vitamin P* and Goldsmiths prize the wood as firewood
    (a) *Acacia leucopholea*   (b) *Acacia arabica*
    (c) *Acacia catechu*   (d) *Acacia senegal*

609. *Paper pulp* can be made out of the bark of young branches
    (a) *Acacia leucophloea*   (b) *Acacia catechu*
    (c) *Acacia concinna*   (d) *Acacia arabica*

610. Match the follwing *Fruits*
    (a) Cape gooseberry (1) *Physalis peruviana* (Solanaceae)
    (b) Tomatillo   (2) *Physalis ixocarpa* (Solanaceae)
    (c) Mammey apple (3) *Mammea americana* (Guttiferae)
    (d) Rambutan   (4) *Nephelium lappaceurm* (Sapindaceae)

162

611. Match the following Fruits
    (a) Granadilla   (1) *Passiflora edulis* (Passifloraceae)
    (b) Mangosteen   (2) *Garcinia mangostana* (Guttiferae)
    (c) Longan   (3) *Hiphoria longan* (Sapindaceae)
    (d) Akee   (4) *Blighia sapida* (Sapindaceae)

612. Which is the lightest of the following woods
    (a) *Cedrus deodara*   (b) *Juniperus virginiana*
    (c) *Thuja occidentalis*   (d) *Pinus roxburghii*

613. Which of the following woods is hard wood or porous wood
    (a) *Cedrus deodara*   (b) *Juniperus virginana*
    (c) *Thuja occidentalis*   (d) *Pinus roxburghii*

614. Which of the following woods is soft wood or porous wood?
    (a) Rose wood, *Dalbergia latifolia*
    (b) Mango wood, *Mangifera indica*
    (c) Sandal wood, *Santalum album*
    (d) Teak wood, *Tectona grandis*

615. *Indian rosewood (Bombay Blackwood)* is
    (a) *Dalbergia latifolia*   (b) *Dalbergia sissoo*
    (c) *Dalbergia nigra*   (c) *Swietenia mahogany*

616. What are the economic uses of Cork (Obtained from the bark of *Quercus suber, Fagaceae*)
    (a) As stoppers for bottles
    (b) Hats, cigarette tips, baseball centres and mats etc
    (c) As insulating material for refrigerators and cold storages
    (d) In high speed jet planes to reduce vibrations and in sound proofing rooms

617. Which of the following woods is used for the construction of *boats* and *Canoes*
    (a) *Cedrus*   (b) *Thuja*
    (c) *Pinus*   (d) *Juniperus*

618. The structural arrangement of various elements on the surface of the timber?
    (a) Texture   (b) Grain
    (c) Tracheids   (d) Fibres

619. Pores of wood are
    (a) Cross sections of vessels

(b) Cross sections of tracheids

(c) T.L.S. medullary rays

(d) R.L.S medullary rays

620. Which of the following woods is used in making pianos, sporting and atheletic goods and in cars.

(a) Rose wood
(b) Pine wood
(c) Cedar wood
(d) Thuja wood

621. Match the following

(a) Wood dye
(b) Bark dye
(c) Leaf dye
(d) Flower dye

1. *Lawsonia inermis*
2. *Butea frondosa*
3. *Acacia catechu*
4. *Mimusops elengi*

622. Match the following

(a) Root dye
(b) Fruit dye
(c) Seed dye
(d) Bark dye

(1) *Mallotus philippinensis*
(2) *Rubia cardifolia*
(3) *Terminatia tomentosa*
(4) *Bixa orellana*

623. The green dye *Kakrezi* is obtained from

(a) *Acacia arabica*, Mimosaceae
(b) *Mallotus philippinensis*, Euphorbiaceae
(c) *Justicia adhatoda*, Acanthaceae
(d) *Punica granatum*, Punicaceae

624. *Lac* consists of a resinous substance produced by the female insect of *Coccus lacca* which is found on the twigs and branches of

(a) *Ficus religiosa*, Pipal
(b) *Feronia limonea*, Elephant apple
(c) *Acacia nilotica*
(d) *Zizyphus jujuba*, Bel

625. Match the following Drugs

(a) Ophelic acid
(b) Hyoscyamine
(c) Hydoscine
(d) Morphine

(1) *Swertia chirata (Chiretta)*
(2) *Atropa belladona*
(3) *Datura metel*
(4) *Papaver somniferum*

626. Match the following

(a) Bark Tannin

(1) *Rhizophora mucronata*

164   *Question Bank*

    (b) Leaf Tannin   (2) *Uncaria gambier*
    (c) Fruit Tannin   (3) *Quercus macrolepis*
    (d) Root Tannin   (4) *Geranium Wallichianum*

627. Match the following
    (a) Wood Tannin   (1) *Castanea dentata*
    (b) Root Tannin   (2) *Sabal palmetto*
    (c) Bark Tannin   (3) *Cassia fistula*
    (d) Fruit Tannin   (4) *Acacia scorpiodes*

628. Which of the following yield *Bark Tannins*
    (a) Quebracho, *Schinopsis Sp.*, Anacardiaceae
    (b) *Rumex hymenosepalus*, Plygonaceae
    (c) *Dipospyros embryopteris*, Ebenaceae
    (d) *Anogeissus latifolia*, Combretaceae

629. Which of the following yield *Bark Tannins*
    (a) *Acacia scorpioides, Cassia auriculata, Cassia fistula, Casuarina equisetifolia Ceriops tagal.*
    (b) *Acacia decurreus, Elaeodendron glaucum, Lagerstroemia parviflora, Rhizophora mucronata*
    (c) *Shorea robusta, Soymida febrifuga, Terminalia arjuna, Zizyphus hylocarpus*
    (d) *Quercus Sp. Tsuga canadensis Bridelia retusa*

630. Which of the following are *drugs from flowers*
    (a) Chamomile, *Matricaria chamomilla* and *Anthemis nobilis* of Compositae
    (b) Santoniin, *Artemesia cina* of Compositae
    (c) Safron, *Crocus sativus* of Iridaceae
    (d) All these

631. Match the following
    (a) Drug from flowers   (1) *Isabghul*
    (b) Drug from leaves   (2) Senna
    (c) Drug from leaves   (3) Cubebs
    (d) Drug from fruits   (4) *Santonin*

632.* Match the following
    (a) Drug from algae   (1) Chloronycetin
    (b) Drug from fungi   (2) Jalap

(c) Drug from roots   (3) Calpheomin
(d) Drug from Stem   (4) Ephedrine

633. Which of the following are *drugs from seeds*
   (a) Digitalis, *Digitalis purpurea*, Scrophulariaceae
   (b) Winter green, *Gaultheria fragrantissima*, Ericaceae
   (c) Vitex, *Vitex negundo*, Verbenaceae
   (d) Quassia, *Quassia amara* and *Picrasma excelsa*, Simarubaceae

634. Which of the following are *drugs from roots*
   (a) Liquorice, *Glycyrrhiza* glabra, Leguminosae
   (b) Senaga, *Polygala Senaga*, Polygalaceae
   (c) Jalap. *Exogonium purga*, Convolvulaceae
   (d) Chiretta, *Swertia chirata*, Gentianaceae

635. What are the economic uses of *Kuth* (Kaliziri) obtained from the roots of *Saussurea lappa* and *S. candicans* of Compositae
   (a) Used as a protective for shawls against insects
   (b) For cure of asthma, Skin diseases
   (c) In perfumery (*pachuk* of commerce), hair oils
   (d) Used as an insecticide Roots do not tarnish, gold braids and embroidery on woolen clothes.

636. Fruits of which of the following plants are used in making *alcoholic beverages.*
   (a) *Elaeagnus multiflora*, Elaeagnaceae
   (b) *Zizyphus abyssinica*, Rhamnaceae
   (c) *Prosopis nigra, P. pubescens*, Leguminosae
   (d) *Sclerocarya caffra, S. schweinfruthii*, Anacardiaceae

637. Rhizomes and roots of *Piper methysticum*, Piperaceae are used in making a *beverage* that relaxed body and mind, induced refreshing sleep, and eased pain
   (a) Kava   (b) Cola
   (c) Chat   (d) Tea

638. What are the economic uses of *Palm Sap*?
   (a) The sap is consumed as a beverage
   (b) Converted into Jaggery
   (c) Converted into vinegar or arak (palm wine)
   (d) Useful for making a cement and imitation of white marble

639. What are the economic uses of *Palm leaves?*
    (a) The leaf-stalk yields the fibre, bassine
    (b) Leaves are made into fans, mats, ola-bags, water baskets, umbrellas, hat etc
    (c) They are useful for thatching; for making paper, for writing upon with an iron stylus; and for manuring rice fields
    (d) All these

640. The gum that exudes from the trunk has adhesive properties; it is used for dressing textiles, and in printing cloth and dyeing
    (a) *Cocos nucifera*   (b) *Annona reticulata*
    (c) *Zea mays*   (d) *Buchnania lanzan*

641. Which of the following are Masticatories?
    (a) Betel leaves   (b) Betel nut
    (c) *Lawsonia* leaves   (d) *Butea* flowers

642. These are the unicellular, epidermal cellulosic hairs which arise from the seed wall
    (a) Flax   (b) Jute
    (c) Coir   (d) Cotton

643. Fibres of secondary phloem
    (a) Flax   (b) Jute
    (c) Moony   (d) Khus

644. *Arhar fibre* is obtained from which part of *Cajanus indica,* Fabaceae
    (a) Leaves   (b) Roots
    (c) Fruits   (d) Stem

645. *Moonj Fibre* is obtained from which part of *Saccharum munja,* Gramineae
    (a) Leaves   (b) Roots
    (c) Fruits   (d) Stem

646. *Baint fibre* is obtained from which part of *Calamus* sp., Arecaceae
    (a) Leaves   (b) Roots
    (c) Fruits   (d) Stem

647. *Sago* starch is obtained from which part of *Metroxylon sago,*
Arecaceae
(a) Grains   (b) Roots
(c) Leaves   (d) Stems

648. *Karaya gum* is obtained from which part of *Sterculia urens,*
Sterculiaceae
(a) Flower   (b) Leaf
(c) Seed   (d) Bark

649. *Chanlmoogra oil* used to cure leprosy, skin diseases, rheumatism, gout and syphilis is obtained from the seeds of
(a) *Nyctanthes arbortristis*
(b) *Gynocardia odorata*
(c) *Hydnocarpus kurzii, H.wightiana*
(d) *Ochrocarpus longifolius*

650. What is the economic importance of *cubebs* (Unripe dired
fruits of *Piper cubeba* of Piperaceae)
(a) Kidney stimulant
(b) Used in the treatment of Catarrah
(c) Diabetes cure
(d) Cancer cure

651. Which of the following are called *Myrobalans*
(a) Fruits of *Terminalia chebula,* Combretaceae
(b) Fruits of *Terminalia bellerica,* Combretaceae
(c) Fruits of *Emblica officinalis,* Euphorbiaceae
(d) All fruits

652. *Alstonia bark, Alstonia scholaris,* Apocynaceae is used
(a) As a substitute of Quinine
(b) As a substitute of chronic dysentry
(c) In the curing liver diseases
(d) In curing respiratory diseases

653. Economic uses of *Cascara bark, Rhamnus purshiana,* Rhamnaceae
(a) In the treatment of uterine disorders
(b) In the treatment of chronic dysentery
(c) Used in the treatment of diarrhoea
(d) Tonic and laxative

654. Match the following
(a) Gum Tragacanth   1. *Acacia senegal*

    (b) Kino gum   2. *Butea frondosa*
    (c) Bengal Kinogum   3. *Pterocarpus marsupium*
    (d) Gum Arabic   4. *Astragalus gummifer*

655. *Shellec resin* used in making sealing wax in paints and polisheds is obtained from
    (a) *Butea monosperma*, Leguminosae
    (b) *Ficus religiosa*, Moraceae
    (c) *Cajanus cajan*, Leguminosae
    (d) *Zizyphus juguba*, Rhamnaceae

656. Match the following
    (a) Para rubber   1. *Hevea brasiliensis, H. benthamiana* Euphorbiaceae
    (b) Panama rubber   2. *Castilla esastica, Moraceae*
    (c) Ceara rubber   3. *Manihot glaziovii, Euphorbiaceae*
    (d) India rubber   4. *Ficus elastica, Moraceae*

657. Match the following
    (a) Lagos Silk Rubber   1. *Funtuma elastica*, Apocynaceae
    (b) Landolphia Rubber   2. *Landolphia Kirkii*, Apocyanaceae
    (c) Guayule Rubber   3. *Parthenium argentatum*, Compositae
    (d) Dandelion Rubber   4. *Taraxacum Koksaghyz*, Compositae

658. Match the following Resins
    (a) Sal damar   1. *Shorea robusta* Diperocarpaceae
    (b) White damar   2. *Vateria indica*, Dipterocarpaceae
    (c) Black damar   3. *Canarium strictum* Burseraceae
    (d) Shellec   4. *Butea monosperma* Legunninosea

659.

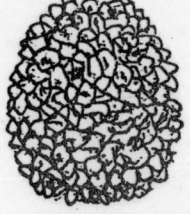 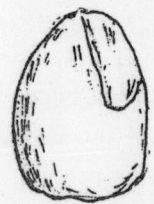

                    A   B

In the above diagram A is the nut of *Litchi chinensis*; B is
    (a) Aril   (b) Aril enclosing the seal
    (b) Seed   (d) Nut in section

660. In the L.S. of Castor Oil seed testa, tegmen, radical and plumule are seen; 2 paery thin cotyledons are pesent, endosperm well developed. In a T.S. of caster oil seed which of the above mentioned parts are not seen
    (a) Endosperm   (b) Radical
    (c) Plumue   (d) Testa and tegmen

661. What are the parts present in a T.S. of Lemon peeling
    (a) Single layered epidermis
    (b) Cortex many layered
    (c) Sub-epidermal essential oil glands
    (d) Each gland consists of a cavity and a glandular epithelium

662. Drugs from *Bark*:
    (a) Quinine   (b) Ashoka
    (c) Cascara   (d) Cinnamon

663. Match the following:
    (a) Cascara   1. *Rhamuus purshiana*
    (b) Cassia   2. *Cinnamomium tamala*
    (c) Ashoka bark   3. *Saraca Indica*
    (d) Kachnar bark   4. *Bauhinia variegata*

664. *Podophyllum hexandrum, giriparpat*, rhizome usefull in constipation, many skin diseass and tumorous growths (curing cancerous tissue) belongs to the Family.
    (a) Orchidaceae   (b) Liliaceae
    (c) Araliaceae   (d) Berberidaceae

665. The resin *ral* imported into India from Singapore, is obtained from
    (a) *Dalbergia sissoo*, Fabaceae
    (b) *Dalbergia latifolia*, Fabaceae
    (c) *Salmalia malabarica*, Malvaceae
    (d) *Shorea robusta*, Dipterocarpaceae

666. Economic uses of ral (*sal dammar, dhooma*) a dark brown to pale amber resin, soluble in alchoid, either and oil of turpentive
    (a) Plasters and ointments for fractures and rheumatism
    (b) Used in blood diarrhoea and dysentery and bleeding piles

(c) As drops in ear trouble, given for weak digestion and leucorrhoea

(d) Fumigating rooms occupied by the Sick

667. The dye obtained by boiling saw dust of the wood of *Jack fruit tree, Artocarpus heterophyllus,* Moraceae
   (a) Kamela   (b) Orchil
   (c) Saffron dye   (d) Basanti

668. A favourite wood for *muscial instruments*
   (a) Jack fruit tree, *Artocarpus heterophyllus,* Moraceae
   (b) Ainiwood tree, *Artocarpus hirsuta,* Moraceae
   (c) Teak *Tectona grandis,* Verbenaceae
   (d) Chaphash, *Artocarpus chaplasha* Moraceae

669. *Margosa of Oil* of commerce is obtained from the seeds of
   (a) *Balnites aegyptiaca,* Simarubiaceae
   (b) *Melia azedarch,* Meliaceae
   (c) *Terminalia chebula,* combretaceae
   (d) *Azadirachta indica,* Meliaceae

670. *Zachun oil* is obtained from the seeds of
   (a) *Melia azedarach,* Meliaceae
   (b) *Swietenia mahogani,* Meliaceae
   (c) *Balanites aegyptiaca,* Simarubaceae
   (d) *Xylocarpus moluccensis,* Meliaceae

671. Economic uses of *margosa oil*
   (a) Manufacuture of soaps, cosmetics
   (b) Disinfectants, emulsifiers; in some pharmaceutical prepartions
   (c) As a luminant
   (d) Insecticidies

672. The *oil cake* is a good substitute for *pyridine* and other agents used in the manufacture of alcohol denaturants
   (a) Cederala Oil   (b) Zachunm Oil cake
   (c) Agaia oil   (d) Neem oil cake

673. *Benzoic acid* is present in the
   (a) Shoots of *Bambusa*
   (b) Shoots of *Cynodon dautylon*
   (c) Shoots of *Saccharum munja*

(d) Shoots of *Chloris barbata*

674. It is in great demand in the manufacutre of good quality
paper pulp
- (a) *Bambusa bambos*
- (b) *Bambusa tulda*
- (c) *Cynodon dactylon*
- (d) *Dactyloctenium sp.*

675. A yellow dye used in the manufacture of *Morocco leather* is
obtained from
- (a) *Lawsonia inermis*, Lythraceae
- (b) *Punica granatum*, Punicaceae
- (c) *Woodfordia fruticosa*, Lythraceae
- (d) *Berberis aristata*, Berberidaceae

676. *Zirishk turash* of commerce are the dried berries of
- (a) *Ammania baccifera*, Lythraceae
- (b) *Duabanga grandiflora*, Lythraceae
- (c) *Sonneratia apetala*, Lythraceae
- (d) *Berberis aristata*, Berberidaceae

677. *Rasut*, a brown extract obtained from the roots and lower
parts of the stem of
- (a) *Heritiera fomes*, Sterculiaceae
- (b) *Guazuma ulmifolia*, Sterculiaceae
- (c) *Melochia corchorifolia*, Sterculiaceae
- (d) *Berberis aristata*, Berberidaceae

678. Extract known as *rasanjan* is obtained from
- (a) *Abroma angusta*, Sterculiaceae
- (b) *Corchorus capsularis*, Tiliaceae
- (c) *Tilia platyphylla*, Tiliaceae
- (d) *Berberis aristata*, Berberidaceae

679. *Dasamula* (10 roots) used in Ayurvedic medicine are
- (a) *Premna integrifolia* (agnimantha), *Aegle marmelos*
(bilwa)*Gmelina arborea* (gambhari)
- (b) *Tribulus terrestris* (gokshura), *Solanum surattense*
(Kantakari), *Terminalia chebula* (haritaki)
- (c) *Sterospermum suaveolens* (patla), *Uraria lagopoides*
(prisniparni), *Desmodium gangeticum* (salparni)
- (d) *Oroxylum indicum* (Syonaka)

680. Timber is suitable for *aircraft* work.
    (a) *Artocarpus hirsuta*, aini, Moraceae
    (b) *Artocarpus heterophyllus*, phanas, Moraceae
    (c) *Artocarpus chaplasha*, Chaplash, Moraceae
    (d) *Artocarpus lakoocha*, Barhal, Moraceae

681. *Dye* is extracted from which of the following parts of monkey fruit, *Artocarpus lakoocha*, Moraceae
    (a) Wood   (b) Roots
    (c) Fruits   (d) Leaves

682. The pulp of the stem and the leaves is suitable for the manufacture of *high grade* writing *paper* and *rayon*.
    (a) *Cynodon dactylon*, Gramineae
    (b) *Chloris barbata*, Gramineace
    (c) *Calamus rotang*, ratan cane, Palmae
    (d) *Arundo donax*, baranal, Gramineae

683. Industrial uses of *ral* (sal dammar, dhooma) an aromatic oleoresinous gum from *Shorea robusta*
    (a) Incense and fumigant; manufacture of inferior quality paints and varnishes
    (b) Carbon papers, type writer ribbons
    (c) Used for caulking boats
    (d) For hardening soft wax used in the manufacture of shoe polishes

684. *Chua oil* used in the manufacture of perfumes and incenses, is distilled from
    (a) Sal butter   (b) Sal dammar
    (c) Sal bark   (c) Sal flowers

685. Economic uses of *tamarind* (*imli*) seeds
    (a) Seeds are rich in the *pectine jellose* which is extensively used in jam and jelly industries.
    (b) The processed seed oil is used as a varnish for painting images and idols
    (c) A cement is made by mixing seed powder with glue. The cement is used for sizing country made blankets
    (d) All these

686. In Bengal, it is much used in cooking as a flavouring agent
    (a) *Carum copticum*, ajwain

(b) *Foeniculum vulgare,* fennel

(c) *Apium graveolens,* ajmod

(d) *Trachyspermum roxburghianum,* ajmod

687. Liquor fermented from *emblic myrobalan (Emblica officinalis)* is good for

(a) Indigestion; Jaundice   (b) Anaemia; cold in nose

(c) For promoting urinatia   (d) Certain heart complaints

688. *Emblic myrobalan* seeds contain

(a) Phosphatides   (b) Fixed oil

(c) Essential Oil   (d) All these

689. Tartaric acid (5 per cent), potassium tartrate (8 per cent) are present in the fruits of

(a) Mango   (b) Jamun

(c) Pomegranate   (d) Tamarind

690. Seeds are an effective drug in thread *worm infection*

(a) *Coriandrum sativum,* Coriander

(b) *Trachyspermum roxburghianum,* ajmod

(c) *Centratherum anthelminticum,* purple fleabane

(d) All these

691. Introduced from Iran and grown in Kashmir and Western parts of U.P.

(a) *Salix caprea,* Salicaceae

(b) *Berberis aristata,* Berberidaceae

(c) *Rhamnus frangula,* Rhamnaceae

(d) *Paliurus aculeatus,* Rhamnaceae

692. *Salix (bed musk)* manna, used in medicine, is found as whitish deposit on

(a) Roots   (b) Fruits

(c) Leaves   (c) Tender twigs

693. Useful for manufacturing *black enamel*

(a) Fruits of marking nut (*Semecarpus anacardium*)

(b) Fruits of cashew nut (*Anacardium occidentale*)

(c) Fruits of *Spondias pinnata*

(d) Fruits of *Rhus parviflora*

694. Indicated in hepatic and spleen enlargement, liver cirrhosis, liver protector against toxic drug and alcohol
    (a) *Tragopogon porrifolium*, Oyster plant, Asteraceae
    (b) *Helianthus tuberosus*, Jerusalem artichoke, Asteraceae
    (c) *Wedelia calendulacea*, Kesaroj, Asteraceae
    (d) *Eclipta alba*, Bhangra, Asteraceae

695. Leaves used as vegetables and as chutneys
    (a) *Tragopogon porrifolium*, Oyster plant, Asteraceae
    (b) *Helianthus tubherosus*, Jerusalem artichoke, Asteraceae
    (c) *Wedelia calendulacea*, Kesaraj Asteraceae
    (d) *Elipta alba*, bhangra, Asteraceae

696. *Uscharin, uscharidin* useful for cardiac principles are obtained from
    (a) *Hemidesmus indicus*, Asclepiadacae
    (b) *Calotropis gigantea*, Asclepiadaceae
    (c) *Calotropis procera*, Asclepiadaceae
    (d) *Asclepias curassivica* Asclepiadaceae

697. It is very useful in *uterine affections* and especially in menorrhagia
    (a) *Cassia fistula*, amaltas
    (b) *Cassia occidentalis*, Kasunda
    (c) *Parkinsonia aculeata* Vilayati Kikar
    (d) *Saraca Indica*, ashok

698. *Bone setter*, applied in fractures of bones
    (a) *Asclepias curassavia*, Asclepiadaceae
    (b) *Proraclea corylifolica*, Fabaceae
    (c) *Cissus quadrangularis*, Vitaceae
    (d) *Viola odorata*, Violaceae

699. *Fermentation of toddy* made effective by
    (a) Pipal bark   (b) Neem bark
    (c) Barged bark   (d) Babul bark

700. Plant which cures *lecodermae* disease
    (a) *Psoralen corylifolia*, Fabaceae
    (b) *Viola odorata*, Violaceae
    (c) *Parkinsonia aculeata*, Caesalpiniaceae
    (d) *Cynodon dactylon*, Gramineae

701. Roots, leaves and blossom contain methyl *salicylate* in the form of a glucoside.
    (a) *Viola odorata*, Violaceae
    (b) *Salix caprea*, Salicaceae
    (c) *Hybanthus enneaspermus*
    (d) *Leonia glycycarpa*, Violaceae

702. Enzyme salicinase is present in
    (a) Bark of *Hybanthus enneaspermus*
    (b) Bark of *Salix caprea*
    (c) Bark *Leonia glycycarpa*
    (d) Bark of *Viola odorata*

703. *The gum Bengal Knol* used as a substitute for the genuine Kno of commerce is obtained from
    (a) *Acacia Senegal*
    (b) *Astragalus gummifer*
    (c) *Pterocarpus marsupium*
    (d) *Butea frondosa*, dhak

704. A durable *blue dye* is obtained from which part of Butea Frondosa
    (a) Flowers   (b) Seeds
    (c) Wood   (d) Gum

705. The flowers are a constituent of *gulal or abir* the powder popularly used at the time of holi or *doljatra festival*
    (a) *Ochrocarpus longifolius*   (b) *Mallotus philippinensis*
    (c) *Butea frondosa*   (d) *Nyctanthes arbortristis*

706. The wood resembles ivory, used for drawing mathematical and musical instruments, fine cabinet work, best Quality combs etc.
    (a) *Casuarina equisetifolia*, Casuarinaceae
    (b) *Dalbergia sissoo*, Shisham, Lequminosae
    (c) *Azadirachta indica*, neem, Meliaceae
    (d) *Buxus wallichiana*, boxwood tree, Buxaceae

707. One of the richest *tannin* bearing trees of Asia
    (a) *Caesalpinia coriaria*, Caesalpiniacae
    (b) *Butea monosperma*, Leguminosae
    (c) *Shorea robusta*, Dipterocarpaceae
    (d) *Canarium strictum*, Burseaceae

708. *Red wood or Brazil wood* (bakam wood) of commerce
   - (a) *Caesalpinia digyna*
   - (b) *Caesalpinia sappan*
   - (c) *Caesalpinia coriaria*
   - (d) *Shorea robusta*

709. The Charcoal made out of the wood is used in gun powder and fire works
   - (a) *Calotropis gigantea*, Asclepiadaceae
   - (b) *Calotropis procera*, Asclepiadaceae
   - (c) *Hemidesmus indicus*, Asclepiadaceae
   - (d) *Anthemis nobilis*, Compositae

710. The well known *perfume* obtained from the first distillation of the flowers of *Canangium odoratum*, Annonaceae
   - (a) Ylang-Ylang
   - (b) Canaga Oil
   - (c) Macassar Oil
   - (d) Sandal Oil

711. The *perfume* obtained from the Second distillation of the flowers of *Canangium odoratum*, Annonaceae
   - (a) Ylang-ylang oil
   - (b) Macassar oil
   - (c) Rose Oil
   - (d) Sandal Oil

712. A substitute for *Burgandy* pitch used in making medical plasters
   - (a) Gum of *Canarium strictum*, Burseraceae
   - (b) Gum of *Astragulus gummifer*, Leguminosae
   - (c) Gum of *Sterculia urens*, Sterculiaceae
   - (d) Gum of *Pterocarpus marsupium*, Leguminosae

713. Which gum is called *Black dammar* of South India
   - (a) Gum of *Canarium strictum*, Burseraceae
   - (b) Gum of *Butea frondosa*, Leguminosae
   - (c) Gum of *Acacia arabica*, Leguminosae
   - (d) Gum of *Acacia senegal*, Leguminosae

714. Wood which can be used for parts of *aeroplanes* and gliders, particularly for Spares.
   - (a) *Canarium strictum*, black damar
   - (b) *Canarium euphyllum*
   - (c) *Canarium odoratum*
   - (d) *Vateria indica*, white damar

715. The red pulp of the fruit is used for colouring cotton wood, silk, butter, cheese, confectionery, hair oils, shoe polishes,

floor polisheds and *pharmaceutical ointments.*

(a) *Punica granatum,* anar, Punicaceae

(b) *Fagonia cretica, damahan,* Zygophyllaceae

(c) *Bixa orellana,* Sendri, Bixaceae

(d) *Pelargonium graveolens,* Geraniaceae

716. The fibre is particularly useful for making paper pulp required for the manufacture of *bank notes*

(a) *Eucalyptus Sp.* Myrtaceae

(b) *Corchorus capsularis,* Tiliaceae

(c) *Tilia platyphylla,* Tiliaceae

(d) *Boehmeria nivea,* Urticaceae

717. Scrapal and hand cleaned ribbons of ramie *fibre* is called

(a) Ramie ribbon   (b) China grass

(c) Ramie wool   (d) Boehmeria ribbon

718. One of the best woods for *match boxes* and match splints

(a) *Bombax malabaricum,* Semal, Bombaceceae

(b) *Dalbergia latifolia,* rosewood, Leguminosae

(c) *Thuja occidentalis,* Gymnosperm

(d) *Juniperus Virginiana,* Gymnosperm

719. The gum-oleo-resin sold in bazaars as *luban or Kundu,* is obtained from

(a) *Sterculia urens,* Sterculiaceae

(b) *Pterocarpus marsupium,* Legumniosae

(c) *Canarium Strictum,* Burseraceae

(d) *Boswellia serrata,* Burseraceae

720. A good substitute for *Pyridine* and other agents used in the manufacture of alcohol denaturants

(a) Neem Oil cake   (b) Sesamum oil cake

(b) Malwa oil cake   (d) Karanj oil cake

721. The flowers are used as pot herb and the leaves as *fodder*

(a) *Bauhinia purpurea, Khairwal,* Lalkachnar

(b) *Bauhnia variegata,* mountain ebony

(c) *Bauhinia vahlii,* Chambuli, mahul

(d) *Parkinsonia aculeata,* Vilayati Kikar

722. At is very valuable for *air-craft* plywood

(a) *Betula utilis,* bhijipattra, Indian paper birch

(b) *Berrya cordifolia*, Chavandalai, Trincomalae wood

(c) *Bischofia javanica*, panialoa Euphorbiaceae

(d) *Betula alnoides*, Khujpattra, Indian birch

723. Used in the manufacture of *Russian leather*
     (a) Bark of *Betula alnoides*   (b) Bark of *Cassia ula*
     (c) Bark of *Betula utilis*   (d) Bark of *Saraca indica*

724. The climbing stem is used for making supension bridges in the Himalayas
     (a) *Calamus rotang*, *retar*, retan cane
     (b) *Bauhina purpurea*, Kachnar
     (c) *Poinciana regia*, gulmohar
     (d) *Bauhinia vahlii*, *Jallur*, mahul

725. Wood is hard and durable when in contact with water, in great demand for *railway sleepers, bridges*, boats
     (a) *Bischofia Javanica*, paniala (b) *Tectona grandis*, Teak
     c) *Shorea robusta*, Sal   (d) *Dalbergia sissoo*, Shisham

726. *Olibanum or frankencense* of the ancients is the gum that exudes from the tree
     (a) *Sterculia urens*, Karaya gunl tree
     (b) *Boswellia serrata*, Sallaki
     (c) *Pterocarpus marsupium*, Kino gum tree
     (d) *Butea frondosa*, Bengal Kno gum tree

727. Used as a substitute of *American pine turpentine*
     (a) Essential oil of olibanum (b) Rosin of olibanum
     (c) White damar   (d) Sal damar

728. Wood used in *railway sleepers and carriages, boat building* etc
     (a) *Eucalyptus Sp.*, Myrtaceae
     (b) *Calophyllum eletum*, poon spar tree, Guttiferae
     (c) *Calophyllum inophyllum*, Alexandrian laurel, Guttiferae
     (d) *Psidium guajava*, Myrtaceae

729. *Tacamahca gum*, an aromatic gum that exudes from the bark of
     (a) *Calophyllum eletum*
     (b) *Calophyllum inophyllum*
     (c) *Astragalus gummifer*, tragacanth
     (d) *Acacia Senegal*, Senegal

730. *Piney or dilo* oil used for soap making and as luminant, is obtained from the seeds of
    (a) *Calophylum eletum,* nagani
    (b) *Calophyllum inophyllum,* punnaga
    (c) *Calophyllum tomentosum,* Poon spar
    (d) All these

731. The manna *madar-ka-shakar* is obtained from
    (a) *Calophyllym inophyllum*   (b) *Calotropis procera*
    (c) *Calotropis gigantea*   (d) *Hemidesmus indicus*

732. Match the follwing
    (a) Neroli bigarade   1. *Citrus aurantium var bigaradia*
    (b) Neroli Portugal Oil   2. *Citrus sinensis*
    (c) Maulsiri Oil   3. *Mimusops elengi*
    (d) Chua oil   4. *Shorea robusta*

733. Match the following
    (a) Petitagrain Oil   1. *Cymbopagon nardus*
    (b) Patcholi Oil   2. *Cinnamomum tamla,*
        C. Cassia
    (c) Cassia Oil   3. *Pogostemon cablin,*
        P. heyeanus
    (d) Citronella oil   4. *Citrus aurantium, C. sinensis*

734. Lemon grass oil is obtained from the leaves of
    (a) *Cymbopogon nardus,* Gramineae
    (b) *Cymbopogon citratus,* Gramineae
    (c) *Cymbopogon martinii,* Gramineae
    (d) *Cymbopogon flexuosus,* Gramineae

735. Kuth oil is obtined from the roots of
    (a) *Cyperus rotundus,* Cyperaceae
    (b) *Acorus calamus,* Araceae
    (c) *Saussurea lappa,* Compositae
    (d) *Curcuma zedoaria,* Zingiberaceae

736. Nair oil is obtained from the leaves of
    (a) *Pelargonium graveolens,* Geraniaceae
    (b) *Pelargonium odoratissimum,* Geraniaceae
    (c) *Santalum album,* Santalaceae
    (d) *Skimmia lureola,* Rutaceae

737. *Loquat (lokath) Eriobotrya japonica*, Rosaceae is a
    (a) Pome fruit   (b) Drupe fruit
    (c) Gourd fruit   (d) Berry fruit

738. Edible portion of *litchi (leechee), Litchi chinensis*, Sapindaceae
    is
    (a) Pericarp   (b) Seed
    (c) Aril   (d) Cotyledons

739. Botanical name of *sweet orange,* Santra
    (a) *Citrus medica lumia*, Rutaceae
    (b) *Citrus limon*, Rutaceae
    (c) *Citrus aurantium*, Rutaceae
    (d) *Citrus sinensis*, Rutaceae

740. Which of the following is a berry fruit
    (a) Banana, *Musa sapientum*, Musaceae
    (b) Pine apple, *Ananas comosus*, Bromeliacaeae
    (c) Melon, *Cucumis melo*, Cucurbitaceae
    (d) Mango, *Mangifera indica*, Anacardiaceae

741. Match the following data on occurrence essential of oils in
    plant parts
    (a) Cardamom 1. Wood   (b) Cinnamon 2. Seeds
    (c) Mint   3. Bark   (d) Cedar   4. Leaves

742. *Cajeput oil* is obtained from the leaves of
    (a) *Cymbopogon nardus*, Gramineae
    (b) *Syzygium aromaticum*, Myrtacaea
    (c) *Melaleuca leucadendron*, Myrtaceae
    (d) *Dianthus caryophyllus*, Caryophyllaceae

743. *Reserpine* the alkaloid employed against hypertension is
    obtained commercially from
    (a) *Rauvolfia serpentina, R. vomitoria*
    (b) *Rauvolfia canescens, R. micrantha, R. tetraphylla, R. caffra,
        R. cubana, R. cumminsii, R. densiflora, R. heterophylla,
        R.hirsuta, R. indecora, R. lamarckii, R. mollis, R. mombasiana,
        R. natalensis, R. obscura, R. perakensis, R. sarapiquensis, R.
        schueli, R. Sellowii*
    (c) *Alstonia constricta, Catharanthus roseus*
    (d) *Tonduzia longifolia, Vinca major*

744. *Antihypertensic agents* are obtained from
    (a) Dried rhizomes and roots of *Veratrum album*
    (b) Seeds of *Schoenocaulon officinalis*
    (c) Dried rhizomes and roots of *Veratrum viride*
    (d) All these

745. *Nuts* with high carbohydrate content
    (a) Chestnut *Castanea vulgaris, C. sativa, C. dentata*
    (b) Acorns, fruits of *Quercus Sp.*
    (c) Coconuit, *Cocos nucifera*
    (d) Cashew nut, *Anacardium occidentale*

746. *Parsnip, Pastinaca sativa*, Umbelliferae is a
    (a) Stem vegetable   (b) Root vegetable
    (c) Fruit vegetable   (d) Green vegetable

747. Which of the following are *above ground vegetables*
    (a) Brussels sprout, *Brassica oleracea var gemmifera*
    (b) Lettuce, *Lactuca sativa*
    (c) Celery, *Apium graveolens*
    (d) Knolkhol, *Brassica oeracea var caulorapa*

748. Which of the following are *pseudocereals*
    (a) Canada rice, *Zizania aquatica*, Gramineae
    (b) Quinoa, *Chenopodium quinoa*, Chenopodiaceae
    (c) Kutu, buck wheat, *Fagopyrum esculentum F. sagittatum* Polygonaceae
    (d) All these

749. *Cowpea* (ramas,, ronsa) is
    (a) *Cajanus cajan*, Fabaceae
    (b) *Glycine soja*, Fabaceae
    (c) *Cicer arietinum*, Fabaceae
    (d) *Vigna sinensis*, Fabaceae

750. *Sieva bean* (lobia) is
    (a) *Phaseolus lanatus*, Fabaceae
    (b) *Phaseolus radiatus*, Fabaceae
    (c) *Phaseolus vulgaris*, Fabaceae
    (d) *Phaseolus mungo*, Fabaceae

751. Green gram of India *(moong)*
    (a) *Phaseolus radiatus*, Fabaceae
    (b) *Phaseolus vulgaris*, Fabaceae
    (c) *Phaseolus mungó*, Fabaceae
    (d) *Arachis hypogea*, Fabaceae

752. Nut with high protein content ·
    (a) Walnut, *Juglans regia*, J. nigra
    (b) Cashewnut, *Anacardium occidentale*
    (c) Butternut, *Jugalns cinerea*
    (d) Beech nut, *Fagus grandiflora*

753. *Nut* with high fat content
    (a) Pistachionut, *Pistacia vera*
    (b) Almond, *Prunus amugdalus var dulcis*
    (c) Beech nut, *Fagus grandiflora*
    (d) Pine nut *Pinus gerardiana, P. edulis, P. torreyana*

754. Which part of *Pandanus tectorius* (kewra) yields essential oil *(attar)*
    (a) Female inflorescence   (b) Male inflorescence
    (c) Roots   (d) Leaves

755. *Bergamot Oil* is obtained from which part of *Citrus aurantium* var *bergania*
    (a) Flowers   (b) Leaves
    (c) Twigs   (d) Fruit rind

756. Which of the following are *scented oils* obtained from flowers
    (a) Lavender oil   (b) Jasmine oil
    (c) Violet oil   (d) Ylang Ylang Oil

757. Which part of *Shorea robusta* of Dipterocarpaceae yields *Chua Oil* used in perfumery
    (a) Stem   (b) Flowers
    (c) Seeds   (d) Leaves

758. Which of the following are *Fruit Spices?*
    (a) Capsicum, black pepper, long pepper
    (b) Nutmeg
    (c) Bishop's weed, cumin, fennel, coriander
    (d) All these

759. Which of the following is a *Flower bud* Spice
    (a) Asafoetida, *Ferula foetida*
    (b) Maulsiri, *Mimusops elengi*
    (c) Saffron, *Crocus sativus*
    (d) Cloves, *Syzygium aromaticum,*

760. Which of the follwing is a *Bark Spice*
    (a) Turmeric, *Curcuma longa, C. domestica*
    (b) Assafoetida, *Ferula foetida and F. narthex*
    (c) Nutmeg, *Myristica fragrans*
    (d) Cinnamon, *Cinnamomum zeylanicum*

761. The true *dalchini* or cinnamon of commerce is obtained from which part of *Cinnamomum zeylanicum*, Lauraceae
    (a) Inner bark of roots   (b) Leaves
    (c) Berries   (d) Inner bark of shoots

762. Camphor (*Kurz*) is obtained from which part of *Cinnamomum zeylanicum*, Lauraceae
    (a) Root bark   (b) Shoot bark
    (c) Leaves   (d) Berries

763. *Cinnamon suet* is the oil extracted from the
    (a) Root   (b) Shoot
    (c) Leaves   (d) Berries

764. *Katira or Hog gum* of commerce, used as a substitute for tragacanth in calico printing, marbliing paper and leather dressing, cosmetics, book binding, shoe making, polish to tusser silk and for thickening ice-creams. The gum is obtained from the trunk of
    (a) *Cochlospermum reliqiosum*, yellow silk cotton tree, Cochlospermaceae
    (b) *Sterculia companulata*, Sterculiaceae
    (c) *Zygophyllum simplex*, alethi, Zygophyllaceae
    (d) *Fagonia cretica, damahax,* Zygophyllaceae

765. The grain is a staple article of diet of the hill and aboriginal tribes of Madhya Pradesh, Sikkim and Assam
    (a) *Paspalum distichum,* Gramineae
    (b) *Iseilema laxum,* Gramineae
    (c) *Eragrostis pilosa,* Gramineae
    (d) *Coix lachryma-jobi,* Gramineae

766. A malted beer called Dzu is prepared from the fermented grain
    (a) *Oryza sativa*, Gramineae
    (b) *Sorghum vulgare*, Gramineae
    (c) *Pennisetum typhoides*, Gramineae
    (d) *Coix lachryma - jobi*, Gramineae

767. *Carob gum or Tragsasol gum* is used for sizing yarns, finishing, painting and back-filling of fabrics as a thickener for colour pastes in calico printing; as a retarder in tanning; used in paper industry; cosmetic prepartions. Carob gum is obtained from which part of *Ceratonia siliquea*, locust tree, Leguimnosae
    (a) Bark   (b) Leaves
    (c) Wood   (d) Seeds

768. What are the economic uses of *Ceriops tagal* a mangrove of Rhizophoraceae
    (a) Wood is used for the kneees of boats, house boats pit props
        and fuel
    (b) All parts of the plant are used in tanning. Sole leather prepared with this tan is very durable
    (c) Bark yields a dye which gives a good black and purple colour with indigo
    (d) Fishing nets are dyed with this bark

769. Wood is used in boats, *railway carriages*. railway sleepers, mathematical instruments, oil mills
    (a) *Ceriops tagal*, Rhizophoraceae
    (b) *Ceratonia siliqua*, Leguminosae
    (c) *Chloroxylon swietenia*, Meliaceae
    (d) *Chukrasia tabularis*, Meliaceae

770. The wood called *Nepal camphor* is obtained from
    (a) *Cinnamomum cecidodaphne*, Lauraceae
    (b) *Cinnamomum tamala*, Laraceae
    (c) *Cinnamomum zeylanicum*, Lauraceae
    (d) *Cinnamomum camphor*, Lauraceae

771. Which part of *cinnamomum tamala* is called Tejpat
    (a) Bark   (b) Roots
    (e) Fruits   (d) Leaves

772. The dye *gunari* used for dyeing cotton and wool fabrics yellow, is obtained from the flowers of
   (a) *Azadirachta indica,* neem, Meliaceae
   (b) *Swietenia mahogani,* mahogany, Meliaceae
   (c) *Melia azedarach, bankayan,* Meliaceae
   (d) *Cedrela toona, toon,* Meliaceae

773. The wood is in great demand as *fuel*
   (a) *Walsura pisidia,* Meliaceae
   (b) *Zizyphus juguba,* Rhammaceae
   (c) *Acer oblongum,* Sapindaceae
   (d) *Casuarina equisetifolia,* Casuarina:eae

774. *Oil* obtained by destructive distil.ation of *Cedrus* wood; used for preserving inflated skins employed for crossing rivers; used in Veterinary medicine
   (a) Cedar wood oil   (b) Cedar leaf oil
   (c) Cedar seed oil   (d) Deodar tar oil

775. *Timber* used in railway sleepers railway carriages, keys of Indian muscial instruments, bri.lge construction
   (a) Deodar wood *Cedrus deodara,* Pinaceae
   (b) Rose wood, *Dalbergia latifolia,* Leguminosae
   (c) Brazilian rose wood, *Dalbergia nigra,* Leguminosae
   (d) Sal, *Shorea robusta,* Dipetrocarpaceae

776. Which of the following are *correct*
   (a) Kapok of commerce is the silky floss covering the seed of *Ceiba pentandra, Bombacaceae*
   (b) Seed oil of *Ceiba pentandra* is used as a food, luminant and in making soaps
   (c) Bark fibre is used in making paper
   (d) Kapok floss is one of the best insulators for heat and sound; used in aeroplane cabins, refrigerators, cold storage plants.

777. The milky juice (latex) of *Calotropis gigantea,* contains
   (a) Cellulolytic enzymes   (b) Proteolytic enzymes
   (c) Amylases   (d) Pectinases

778. *Bar,* an intoxicating liquor, and *Giya,* a ferment are preapred from the latex of
   (a) *Calotropis gigantea,* Asclepiadaceae

(b) *Argemone mexicana*, Papaveraceae
(c) *Euphorbia tirucalli*, Euphorbiaceae
(d) *Nerium odorum*, Apocynaceae

779. The *charcoal* made out of the wood of *Calotropis* is used in
(a) Gun powder   (b) Fire works
(c) Agricultural implements   (d) Boat Knees

780. Which of the following can be prepared from the silky *floss* of seed of *Calotropis*
(a) Shawls and handkerchiefs   (b) Paper
(c) For stuffing pillows   (d) All these

781. Important uses of Carallia wood, *Carallia barachiata*, Rhizophoraceae
(a) Railway carriages
(b) Agricultural implements
(c) Rice pounders, cabinet making
(d) Flooring, staircases

782. The *oil* extracted from the seeds of *Carallia brachiata*, panasi is used as
(a) Cooking medium   (b) Medicine for ringworm
(c) Warnish and in paints   (d) Shoepolish

783. The leaves are used for making bidis, Burma cheroots and for feeding tassar silk worms
(a) *Careja arborea*, Lecythidaceae
(b) *Carallia brachiata*, Rhizophoreceae
(c) *Carica papaya*, Caricaceae
(d) *Carissa carandas*, Apocynaceae

784. What are the *enzymes* present in the Latex of Papaya tree, *Carica papaya*, Caricaceae?
(a) Papain   (b) Chymopapain
(c) Pepsin   (d) Trypsin

785. What are the economic uses of Dried Latex of Papaya tree, *Carica papaya*, Caricaceae
(a) Used in cheese industry because of its mil dotting properties
(b) Used in wool industry
(c) Used in tanning
(d) Used in food, brewing

786. What are the economic uses of leaves of papaya tree, *Carica papaya?*
    (a) Vitamin C is present
    (b) Vitamin E is present
    (c) A glycoside, carposide and an alkaloid carpaine are present
    (d) It can be used as a detergent

787. *Insect repellent* powder is prepared from which part of *Carissa carandas,* Apocynaceae
    (a) Wood   (b) Roots
    (c) Berries   (d) Leaves

788. This oil is usefull as a strong *cement for galss* and stone
    (a) Roghum oil from *Carthamus oxycantha*
    (b) Coconut oil from *Cocos nucifera*
    (c) Cedar wood oil from *Juniperus vigriniana*
    (d) Chua oil from *Shorea robusta*

789. Oil content in *almond kernels* is about
    (a) 400 gm oil per Kg Kernel weight
    (b) 300 gm oil per Kg Kernel weight
    (c) 250 gm Oil per Kg Kernel weight
    (d) No oil is present

790. Which of the following protects membrane damage in Human Cells, caused by environemntal pollutants like *gaseous pollutants, Chemical pollutants and radiation*
    (a) Ergotamin from the ergot fungus *Claviceps*
    (b) Podophyllin from *Podophyllym emodi*
    (c) Capsaicin, the pungent principle of red hot chilli
    (d) Chirating from *Swertia chiraia*

791. Which part of divi-divi, *Caesapinia coriaria* used for *tanning* leather?
    (a) Leaves   (b) Pods
    (c) Wood   (d) Roots

792. The *tannin* in the natural teri pods, *Caesalpinia digyna* is
    (a) Tannic acid   (b) Gallic acid
    (c) Glucose   (d) Monodiallyol glucose

793. *Brazilin,* a dye of red and violet shades from the heartwood

extensively used fro dyeing wood, cotton and silk obtained from

(a) *Caesalpinia coriaria*   (b) *Caesalpinia digyna*

(c) *Cesalpinia sappan*   (d) *Caesalpinia bonducella*

794. *Gulal or Abir*, a powder popularly used on the occasion of Holi or Dojatra festival is obtained from

(a) *Caesalpinia coriaria*   (b) *Caesalpinia digyna*

(c) *Caesalpinia sappan*   (d) *Caesalpinia bonducella*

795. The pods are used in place of Sumach in the tanning of light leather

(a) *Caesalpinia coriaria*   (b) *Caesalpinia digyna*

(b) *Caesalpinia sappan*   (d) *Caesalpinia bonducella*

796. Oil used as *preservative of leather* goods

(a) Safflower oil, *Carthmus tinctorius*

(b) Roghum oil, *Carthmus oxycantha*

(c) Argemone oil, *Argemone mexicana*

(d) Cotton seed oil, *Gossypium sps.*

797. The bark is used for adulterating *Kamela dye*.

(a) *Casearia tomentosa*, Chilla, Flacourtiaceae

(b) *Flacourtia ramontchi*, bowchi, bilangra, Flacourtiaceae

(c) *Flacourtia cataphracta*, Paniala, talispatra, Flacourtiaceae

(d) All these

798. The bark is in great demand for *crust tanning* for *heavy hides (leather)*

(a) *Cassia auriculata*, Leguminosae

(b) *Cassia fistula*, Leguminosae

(c) *Cassia sophera*, Leguminosae

(d) *Cassia occidentalis*, Leguminosae

799. *Sumari bark* of commerce an usefull tanning meterial is obtained from

(a) *Cassia auriculata*, Leguminosae

(b) *Cassia fistula*, Leguminosae

(c) *Cassia sophera*, Leguninosae

(d) *Cassia occidentalis*, Leguminosae

800. The bark is used for dyeing *fishing nets;* for tanning and dyeing leather

(a) *Casuarina equisetifolia*, Casuarinaceae

(b) *Calotropis gigantea*, Asclepiadaceae

(c) *Azadirachta indica*, Meliaceae

(d) *Argemone mexicana*, Papaveraceae

801. Wood suitable for modelling *aircraft*

   (a) Balsa, *Ochroma lagopus; Albizia odoratissima*

   (b) Arjili, *Artocarpus hirsuta; Indian birch, Bejuda*

   (c) Dhup, *Canarium euphyllum, Chikrassy alnoides, Chukrasi tubuolaris*

   (d) Shisham, *Dalbergia latifolia*, Champa, *Michelia Champaca;* padauk, *Petrocarpus indicus*

802. Leaves of which of the following treeds, if boiled with broken rice and leaves of ach (*Morinda citrifolia*), made into a salt gruel, make a good *nutritive* food for children.

   (a) Leaves of *Pongamia pinnata*, Karanj, Fabaceae

   (b) Leaves of *Azadirachta indica*, neem, Meliaceae

   (c) Leaves of *Mangifera indica*, Mango, Anacardiaceae

   (d) Leaves of *Tamarindus indica*, imli, Caesalpiniaceae

803. The leaves of which of the following plants are *edible?*

   (a) *Taraxacum officinale*, dandelion, Compositae

   (b) *Toddalia asiatica*, tindupara, Rutaceae

   (c) *Rumax hastatus*, Khata palak, Polygonaceae

   (d) *Nasturtium officinale*, brachmi sag, water cross, Cruciferae

804. Which of the following members of *Asclepiadaceae* are edible (edible shoots)

   (a) *Caralluma adscendens, Marsdenia volubilis*

   (b) *Caralluma fimbriata*, maked shingi *Leptadenia reticulata*

   (c) *Ceropegia bulbosa*, Khapparkadu; *Tylophora* spp.

   (d) *Gymnema sylenstris*, gurmar; *Holostemma annularis*, chirval

805. *Sabai grass* which yields an excellent pulp for the manufature of printing and medium quality *writing paper*

   (a) *Tragus biflorus*, Gramineae ·

   (b) *Imperata cylindrica*, Gramineae

   (c) *Lolium temulentum*, Gramineae

   (d) *Eulaliopsis binata*, Gramineae

806. Wood is used in *railway keys, railway sleepers* rice pounders, engine break blocks, beaming in *gold fields*, road rammers,

platform boards, setts ladders, etc.

  (a) *Shorea robusta,* Dipterocarpaceae

  (b) *Hibiscus rosa-sinensis,* Malvaceae

  (c) *Hemidesmus indicus,* Asclepiadaceae

  (d) *Hopea parviflora,* Dipterocarpaceae

807. Wood is used in *railway sleepers,* boat builting, roofting, flooring, ship blocks, *caspstan bars, oil* and *sugarcane presses*

  (a) *Hopea odorata,* thingan, Dipterocarpaceae

  (b) *Morus indica,* mulberry, Moraceae

  (c) *Casuarina equisetifolia,* beef wood tree Casuarinaceae

  (d) *Cedrela toona,* toon, Meliaceae

808. Leaves are used for *dyeing* and ias cattle *fodder.*

  (a) *Hymenodictyon ecelsum,* bhaulan, Rubiaceae

  (b) *Anthocephalus indicus,* Kadam, Rubiaceae

  (c) *Cinchona calisaya,* Cinchona, Rubiaceae

  (d) *Randia uliginosa,* Rubiaceae

809. The grass is planted to bind the soil of river banks, railway embankents, dams and coastal sand dumes, and also to reclaim dry and *desert areas*

  (a) *Iseilema laxum*

  (b) *Chrysopogon aciculatus,* love thron

  (b) *Pasaplum distichum*

  (d) *Imperata cylindrica,* dabh

810. The plant is grown in mangrove areas as a mud-binder and land-builder

  (a) *Hibiscus tiliaceus,* bola

  (b) *Hibiscus rosa- sonensis,* gurhal

  (c) *Hibiscus mutabilis,* sthalpadma

  (d) *Hibiscus sabdariffa,* patwa

811. The bark is used for *clarifying sugar cane juice* in gur manufacture

  (a) *Grewia asiatica,* Phalsa, Tiliaceae

  (b) *Guazuma ulmifolia,* Bastard cedar, Sterculiaceae

  (c) *Gossypium herbaceum,* Cotton, Malvaceae

  (d) *Gynandropsis gynandra,* hurhur, Capparidaceae

812. Wood suitable for making *athletic equipment* like horizontal bars, trapeze etc. Sports equipments like *Golf shafts, Billiard cue shafts, Cricket stumps*
    (a) *Corchorus capsularis*, Tiliaceae
    (b) *Triumfetta Sp*, Tiliaceae
    (c) *Grewia tillifolia*, Tiliaceae
    (d) *Sparmannia Sp*, Tiliaceae

813. The wood is extemely hard, very heavy, durable and *resistant* to rot and white ants
    (a) *Hardwickia binata*, Leguminosae
    (b) *Haematoxylon campechianum*, Leguminosae
    (c) *Tamarindus indica*, Leguminosae
    (d) *Xylia xylocarpa*, Leguminosae

814. The oleo-resin that exudes from the stem is valuable as a *wood preservative.*
    (a) *Hardwickia binata*, anan, Leguminosae
    (b) *Pongamia pinnata*, Karanj, Leguminosae
    (c) *Dalbergia sissoo*, Shisham, Leguminosae
    (d) *Dalbergia latifolia*, Sitsal, Leguminosae

815. Conomic uses of common *ginger lilly, Hedychium coronarium, Zingiberaceae*
    (a) Flowers yield a pleasant and elicate perfume
    (b) Rhizome contains starch
    (c) Aerial stems are raw material for paper making. The paper has consierable stength, elasticity and folding qualities
    (d) Sate (*H.specatum*) rhizome is useful in colic, cough, asthma, diarrhoea, dysentery, dropsy, headache, liver complaints

816. Root bark of which plant yields *Chay-root dye* a red, purple, brown orange dyes for calico, wood and silk fabrics
    (a) *Hedychium spicatum*, Zingiberaceae
    (b) *Hedyotis umbellata*, Chiral, Rubiaceae
    (c) *Anthocephalus kadamba*, Kada, Rubiaceae
    (d) *Cephalis ipecacuanha*, Ipecac, Rubiaceae

817. Economic uses of *Helicteres isora*, bhendu, Sterculiaceae
    (a) Fibre from the inner bark is more durable than jute used for making containere bags for rice, arecanuts etc.

(b) Leaves and tender turgs are used as cattle fodder

(c) Stalks are used for the manufacture of printing and writing paper

(d) Fibre is used for making canvas

818. Which part of sundri, *Heritiera minor*, Sterculiaceae are used in the *tanning industry*

(a) Roots   (b) Wood

(c) Leaves   (d) Bark

819. Which of the following are *true*.

(a) The leather treated with sundri leaf tans is of light cream colour but may redden on exposure

(b) The leather treated with Sundri leaf tans is soft, Supple and tough

(c) The leather tanned with sundri bark is reddish buff in colour, tough and supple

(d) All these

820. What are the economic uses of ambari (*Hibiscus cannabinus*, Malvaceae) *seed oil*

(a) Lubricant and illuminant

(b) Usaed for making soaps, linoleum, paints and vanished

(c) Refined oil is edible

(d) All these

821. What are the economic uses of *Excoecaria agallocha*, a mangrove of Euphorbiaceae?

(a) Wood is used for general carpentry, packing cases, togs, bedsteads, tables, floats for fishing nets

(b) Wood is used for match splints of the second quality.

(c) Wood is used for paper pulp; power alcohol manufacture; charcoal; fuel

(d) All these

822. *Wood apple gum* (*Feronia limonia*, Rutaceae) is used

(a) As a substitute for gum arabic

(b) For making artist's water colours

(c) Dyes and varnishes

(d) All these

823. The leaves are used as *fodder* for cattle.

(a) *Ficus glomerata*, gular, Moraceae

(b) *Ficus religiosa*, pipal, Moraceae
(c) *Ficus bengalensis*, bargad, Moraceae
(d) All these

824. Wood is suitable for making *match boxes*
(a) *Ficus glomerata*　　　　(b) *Ficus religiosa*
(c) *Ficus benghalensis*　　　(d) All these

825. Hardened latex is used for filling up cavities in hollow ornaments?
(a) *Ficus glomerata*　　　　(b) *Ficus religiosa*
(c) *Ficus benghalensis*　　　(d) All these

826. The seeds yields an *edible fat*
(a) *Garcinia indica*, Guttiferae
(b) *Garcinia morella*, Guttiferae
(c) *Garcinia mangostana*, Guttiferae
(d) *Garcinia florida*, Guttiferae

827. The chief constituent of *Indian Wintergreen oil (Gaultheria grantissima*, Ericaceae)
(a) Methyl salicylate　　　　(b) Benzoic acid
(c) Ferulic acid　　　　　　　(d) Thymol

828. *Roel or Bhand* root which yields a *red dye* used for colouring medicinal oils, is obtained from
(a) *Geranium ocellatum*,
(b) *Gmelina arborea*
(c) *Geranium nepalense*, Geraniaceae
(d) *Geranium wallichianum*, Geraniaceae

829. Roots yields *tannius* used for tanning *leather*
(a) *Geranium ocellatum*, Geraniaceae
(b) *Pelargonium graveolens*, Geraniaceae
(c) *Geranium nepalense*, Geraniaceae
(d) *Geranium wallichianum*, Geraniaceae

830. *Pearl Ash or Potash salts* are prepared from the wood of
(a) *Gmelina arborea*, Verbenaceae
(b) *Verbena officinalis*, Verbenaceae
(c) *Priva laevis*, Verbenaceae
(d) *Congea tomentosa*, Verbenaceae

831. Which parts of *Gmelina arborea* are used in *Dyeing*
     (a) Wood ash   (b) Drupes
     (c) Leaves   (d) Roots

832. Wood useful for making *musical instruments, stethscopes,*
     match sticks and match boxes?
     (a) *Gmelina arborea,* Verbenaceae
     (b) *Girardiana heterophylla,* urticaceae
     (c) *Grenia asiatica,* Tiliaceae
     (d) *Grewia elastica,* Tiliaceae

833. Match the following
     (a) Wood durable in sea water   *Hibiscus tiliacorus,*
                                          Malvaceae
     (b) Henna + rhizome —> malagiridye *Hedychium spicatum,*
                                          Zingiberaceae
     (c) Bimli jute fibre   *Hibiscus cannabinus,*
                                          Malvaceae
     (d) Cork wood   *Hibiscus tiliaceus,*
                                          Malvaceae

834. *Indian arrowroot* is
     (a) *Hitchenia caulina,* Zingiberaceae
     (b) *Zingiber officinale,* Zingiberaceae
     (c) *Curcuma longa,* Zingiberaceae
     (d) *Costus speciosus,* Zingiberaceae

835. Risinous juice of which plant is use for *waterproofing boats* and
     furniture.
     (a) *Odina wodier,* Jhingan, Anacardiaceae
     (b) *Holigarna arnottiana holgeri,* Anacardiaceae
     (c) *Spondias pinnata,* hogplum, Anacardiaceae
     (d) *Buchanania latifolia, Chirongi,* Anacardiaceae

836. Wood is used for warper bobbins for jute mills, multi-ply jute
     bobbins, cotton reels, *match boxes* and splints, paper pulp etc.
     (a) *Holoptelea integrifolia,* Ulmaceae
     (b) *Trema orientalis,* Ulmaceae
     (c) *Ulmus suberosa,* Ulmaceae
     (d) *Celtis cinnamomea,* Ulmaceae

837. *Rock Dammar* of commerce used for caulking boats, mount-
     ing microscopic objects is the resin of
     (a) *Hopea odorata,* thingan, Dipterocarpaceae

(b) *Shorea robusta*, sal, Dipterocarpaceae

(c) *Dalbergia sissoo*, Shishahu, Leguminosae

(d) *Dalbergia latifolia*, rose wood, Leguminosae

838. Which of the following wood is used in making *Cricket bats*
   (a) *Santalum album*, Sandal wood
   (b) *Sapindus detergens*, Soapnut
   (c) *Saraca indica*, Ashok
   (d) *Salix purpurea*, Willow

839. Economic uses of *lasora, Cordia dichotoma*, Boraginaceae
   (a) Wood used for boat building, agricultural implements, cart building, furniture, fuel etc.
   (b) Bark yields a course fibre used for making cordage paper pulp, for caulking boats.
   (c) Leaves used for wrapping Burma cheroots and for making plates
   (d) Fruits are edible. Spirituous liquors are prepared from the fruit.

840. Which part of *Corypha umbraculifera* fan palm is edible.
   (a) Seeds   (b) Leaves
   (c) Drupe   (d) Pith of trunk

841. *Sumach,* a tannin and dye which is in great demand for tanning soft leather for gloves and book binding; in calico printing etc. Such is obtained from which part of *Cotinus cogygria darengri*, Anacardiaceae
   (a) Dried wood   (b) Dried leaves
   (c) Dried leaf stalks   (d) Dried young branches

842. *Shahi Zafran* of commerce is the
   (a) Three long petals of flower of *Crocus sativus*
   (b) Three long satigvas of flower of *Crocus sativus*
   (c) The red orange tip of stigna of flower of *Crocus sativas*
   (d) The long styles of flower of *Crocus sativus*

843. In India *Hockey sticks* are generally made from the wood of
   (a) *Ficus benghalensis*, Moraceae
   (b) *Streblus asper*, Moraceae
   (c) *Castilla elastica*, Moraceae
   (d) *Morus alba*, Moraceae

844. What are the economic uses of *saffron* obtained from *Crocus sativus, Iridaceae*
    (a) It is used as a dye; blue or green dyes are produced with sulphuric acid or nitric acid or iron sulphate
    (b) With an iron mordant, illuminated manuscripts can be made to resemble gold.
    (c) Used for colouring and flavouring confections, pastry, butter, cheese etc.
    (d) All these

845. *Shoti starch* of commerce used as a substitute for arrowroot and barley is obtained from
    (a) *Curcuma longa*, Zingiberaceae
    (b) *Curcuma Zedoaria*, Zingiberaceae
    (c) *Zingiber officinale*, Zingiberaceae
    (d) *Costus speciosus*, Zingiberaceae

846. Economic uses of *Cyperus rotundus*, mustak Cyperaceae
    (a) Leaves and stems ae fodder for cattle
    (b) The rhizomes are fed to pigs.
    (c) Rhizome oil is used in perfumery, Soaps, agarbatties, for scarting clothes; insect repellent
    (d) Rhizome usefull in appeasing of thirst disorders of stomach; heals urends and ulcers; pain in abdomen and in scorpion stings.

847. It is the most valuable wood for *pencil making*
    (a) *Juniperus macropoda*   (b) *Cedrus deodara*
    (c) *Pinus longifolia*   (d) *Taxus baccata*

848. An oleoresin obtained by tapping the stem, is used as wood varnish; volatile oil from the stem is used as a *substitute for clove oil.*
    (a) *Argemone mexicana*, Papaveraceae
    (b) *Butea monosperma*, Leguminosae
    (c) *Arachis hypogaea*, Leguminosae
    (d) *Kingiodendron pinnatum*, Leguminosae

849. The wood is suitable for *match sticks* and *inside boxes of matches. The leaves* are valued as *fodder*
    (a) *Kydia calycina*, pula, Malvaceae
    (b) *Lagerstroemia lauceolata*, bentcak, Lythraceae

(c) *Hibiscus sabdariffa, Rozelle,* Malvaceae

(d) *Hibiscus cannabinus,* Madras hemp, Malvaceae

850. Match the following

(a) Wood used for shipcorights	*Lagesrtroemia lauceolata benteak* bridges, railway carrigages, motor lorry and bus bodies
(b) Wood used for match splints	*Lagerstroemia speciosa and* and match boxes *L. lanceolata*
(c) Wood used for railway sleepers,	*Lagerstroemia parviflora* wedges for ship's hatches boats carts, water 'tanks
(d) Wood ecellent for ship buildings	*Lagerstroemia speciosa jarul* Canoes; railway carriages; sleepers motor, lorry bodies, water tanks

851. Which of the following tests for tannins are used for testing *tannins* in plant parts

(a) Take a little water extract of the plant material add to it a little *potassium dichromate* solution - a precipitate is obtained.

(b) Add to the extract a little *lead acetate* solution - a precipitate is formed.

(c) Take a little extact in a test tube add a drop of *ferric chloride* solution - a blue or black colour is obtained

(d) Take a little extract in a test tube add a few drops of *potassium ferrocyanide* - it turns deep red in colour.

852. The colour of *Indigo* dye obtained from *Indigofera tinctoria,* Fabaceae

(a) Yellow   (b) Red

(c) Green   (d) Blue

853. *Curcas oil* used in the manufacture of har soap, candles, wood spining and for the manufacture of *Turkey red,* is obtained from the decorticated seeds of

(a) *Croton tiglium,* Jamalgota, Euphorbiaceae

(b) *Croton bonplandianum*, Euphorbiacaeae

(c) *Jatropha curcas*, Physic nut, Euphorbiaceae

(d) *Euphorbia antiquorum*, Bajbaran, Euphorbiaceae

854. Economic uses of *Juglaus regia*, Walnut, Juglandaceae

(a) Wood is used in making aeroplace propeller blades, Indian pipes and hookas

(b) Rind of green fruit is used for staining wood

(c) Bark, leaves and green hulls and shells of nut are used for dyeing and tanning

(d) The Kernel is edible; Kernel oil is used for artists oil colour printingg inks, Soaps and Varnishes.

855. The succulent corollas of *mahua (Madhuca longifolia, M. indica)* are rich in

(a) Calcium   (b) Vitamins

(c) Suga·s   (d) All these

856. Match the following: (regarding Kamala, Mallosus philippinensis, Euphorbiaceae)

(a) Kamala dye   1. Anti-oxidant for ghee, Vegetable oils and shortenings

(b) Kamala seed oil   2. Rapid drying paints and varnishes

(c) Kamala seed oil   3. Insulating boards, cork substitutes Cake + saw dust

(d) Kamala wood   4. Match boxes, cotton reels; fuelwood

857. Which of the following are True?

(a) The dry flower buds of *Mammea longifolia* nag Kesar, Guttiferae dye silk red.

(b) Kamala dye is obtained from the glandular pubescence of the ripe fruit of *Mallotus philippinensis*

(c) Kama dye is used for colouring food - stuffs and beverages

(d) Kamala dye dyes silk and wool yellow or flame colour

858. Match the following regarding the uses of *mango (Mangifera indica, Anacardiaceae)*

(a) Urine of cows fed only on mango leaves 1. Bark dye

(b) Distilled mango flowers   2. Wood

    (c) Cloth dyed blue with indigo change to green

                                         3. Piúry (perirang)

    (d) Masula boats, ploughs, yokes   4. Amb attar

859. What are the economic uses of *bark fibre* of *Marsdenia tenacissima,* rajmahal hemp, *Asclepiadaceae*
    (a) For making bows strings (b) For making cordage
    (c) For making netting   (d) All these

860. The papery bark is resistant to decay; replaces cork as insulating material
    (a) Cajaput tree   (b) Rajmahal hemp
    (c) Madras hemp   (d) Hemp

861. Match the following
    (a) Tennis rackets   1. *Lagerstroemia lanceolata benteak*

    (b) Golf stick shafts   2. *Lagestroemia parviflora*
    (c) Sport goods   3. *Madhuca longifolia M. Indica*

    (d) Sport ware   4. *Melia azedarach*

862. What are the economic uses of *Jhingan gum* (from the bark of *Lannea coromandelica,* Anacardiaceae)
    (a) Clarification of sugar-cane juice; in confectionery
    (b) In the manufacture of inks
    (c) It is mixed with lime for white washing and plastering
    (d) Mixed with dhaura gum, used in calico

863. Match the following (Dyeing of fabrics by *henna leaves, Lawsonia inermis,* Lythraceae)
    (a) Henna + Indigo   1. Black dye
    (b) Henna + catechu   2. Deep red dye
    (c) Cotton dyeing with   3. Light reddish brown
        henna   (malagiri)
    (d) Wool, silk dyeing with 4. Reddish or yellowish
        henna   brown

864. What are the economic uses of *Madhua Seed oil (Madhuca longifolia and M.indica,* Sapotaceae) and Oil cake
    (a) Manufacture of margarine and soap; particularly lanundry soap

(b) Dil is edible; luminant

(c) Oil cake is used as a fertilizer

(d) Oil cake is applied to lawns and golf freen to kill earthworms; used as a detergent for washing hair. *

865. What are the uses of *Madhua wood*?
(a) Used for bridge construction
(b) Ship's keel and planking below the water line
(c) Oil and sugarcane presses
(d) Agricultural implements, muscial instruments

866. *Oil of Cajuput* obtained from *Melaleuca quinquenervia*, Myrataceae used in medicated ointments, liniments; a strong insect repellent is obtained from
(a) Seeds, fruits   (b) Wood
(c) Roots   (d) Leaves, terminal

867. Economic uses of *Persian lilac, Melia azedarach,* Meliaceae?
(a) Wood used for house building, agricultural instruments
(b) Fruits used as insecticides, flea powders
(c) Alcohol can be prepared from the fruit
(d) Seed oil used for making soaps, hair oils.

868. *Otto of Nagkesar* prepared by enfleurage wish olive oil, used in perfuming soaps, is obtained from which part of *Mesua ferrea*, Guttiferae
(a) Flowers   (b) Leaves
(c) Wood   (d) Seeds

869. Match the following
(a) Edible oil from the seeds   1. *Minusops elengi*, Sapotaceae

(b) Camphor from wood   2. *Michelia champaca*, Magnoliaceae

(c) Boats wood used in railway   3. *Mesua ferrea*, sleepers   Guttiferae

(d) Leaf dye - mats and cotton   4. *Memecylon* fabrics   *umbellatum* Melastomaceae

870. *Dye Warrus* which is highly prized for dyeing silk (not suitable for dyeing lineu or cotton) is obtained from which part of *Moghania macrophylla,* Leguminosae
(a) Leaves   (b) Wood
(c) Roots   (d) Pods

871. *Togari* dye obtained from *Morinda coreia*, Rubiaceae (dyes mordanted cotton, silk and wool to shades of red, purple and chocolate) is obtained from which part of the plant?
   (a) Stem Bark   (b) Root bark
   (c) Leaves   (d) Fruits

872. The *root dye of Morinda angustifolia* darnharidra, Rubiaceae stain cotton yarn and cloth
   (a) Yellow   (b) Red
   (c) Chocolate   (d) Purple

873. The *gum of sainjna (Moringa oleifera)* Moringaceae) used in calico printing and as a substitute for tragacanth gum, is obtained from
   (a) Roots   (b) Stem
   (c) Fruits   (d) Seeds

874. Wood is used fro the manufature of *Hockey sticks, Tennis and Badminton rackets, Cricket bats etc.*
   (a) *Morus alba*, Moraceae
   (b) *Ficus benghalensis*, Moraceae
   (c) *Ficus elastica*, Moraceae
   (d) *Ficus religiosa*, Moraceae

875. In which of the following plants, the bark is fragrant and used in the preparation of cosmetics
   (a) *Mucuna pruriens*, Fabaceae
   (b) *Murraya exotica*, Rutaceae
   (c) *Murraya Koenigii*, Rutaceae
   (d) *Murraya Paniculata*, Rutaceae

876. Well known filling material for *life-jacket* and sleeping bags
   (a) *Salmalia malabarica*   (b) *Calotropis procera*
   (c) *Cynodon dactylon*   (d) *Gossypium herbaceum*

877. Antibiotic *pterygospermin* active against gram-positive, gram-negative and acid-fast bacteria is obtained from the leaves of
   (a) *Moringa oleifera*, Sobhangan, Moringaceae
   (b) *Morus alba*, mulberry, Moraceae
   (c) *Musa paradisiaca*, Kela, Musaceae
   (d) *Murraya exotica*, marchula, Rutaceae

878. *Argemone mexicana* seed oil is adulterated with mustar oil for profiteering. Simple test to check the adulteration is to treat with a few drops of nitric acid when the oil turns
    (a) Rich orange red   (b) Rich purple
    (c) Dark brown   (d) Black

879. *Tejpat* leaves are obtained from
    (a) *Cinnamomum tamala*, Lauraceae
    (b) *Cinnamomum macrocarpum*, Lauraceae
    (c) *Cinnamomum obtusifolium*, Lauraceae
    (d) All these

880. Bark given to cattle when suffering from *rinder pest*
    (a) *Ficus racemosa*, gular, Moraceae
    (b) *Ficus religiosa*, Peepal, Moraceae
    (c) *Ficus glomerata*, fig, Moraceae
    (d) *Ficus benghalensis*, bargad, Moraceae

881. Fish leaves cooked as vegetable curry and eatern in stomach and *hepatic troubles*
    (a) *Erythrina variegata*, Fabaceae
    (b) *Dalbergia tamaricifolia*, Fabaceae
    (c) *Clitoria ternatea*, Fabaceae
    (d) *Abrus precatorius*, Fabaceae

882. Dired flowers contain *saccharine*
    (a) *Stereospermum suaveolens*, Bignoniaceae
    (b) *Hibiscus rosa-sinensis*, Malvaceae
    (c) *Mimosa pudica*, Mimosaceae
    (d) *Bauhinia purpurea*, Caesalpiniaceae

883. *Pipla mul (Piper longum)* in combination with borax and baiberang in equal doses used as
    (a) Dye   (b) Contraceptive
    (c) Medicine for skin diseases   (d) Substitute of Coffee

884. Much used in *Veterinary medicine*
    (a) *Inula racemosa*, compositae
    (b) *Parthenium argentatum*, Compositae
    (c) *Chrysanthemum cinerariaefolium*, Compositae
    (d) *Wedelia calendula*, Compositae

885. *Priyangu* sold in Indian baazers are
   (a) Seeds of *Algaia roxburghiana*, Meliaceae
   (b) Seeds of *Callicarpa microphylla*, Verbenaceae
   (c) Seeds of *Verbena officinalis*, Verbenaceae
   (d) Seeds of *Verbena officinalis*, Verbenaceae

886. A resin used for *fumigating rooms* occupied by the sick
   (a) Sal damar from *Shorea robusta*, Dipterocarpaceae
   (b) White damar from *Vateria robusta*, Dipterocarpaceae
   (c) Black damar from *Canarium stricturm*, Dipterocarpaceae
   (d) Shellae from *Zizyphus jujuba*, Rhamnaceae

887. A paste of the root is rubbed on the skin to relieve oppressive
   heat or burning of the body. An *aromatic cooling* bath is
   prepared by adding to a tub of water the roots in fine
   powder, together with the root of *Pavonia odorata*, red sandal-
   wood and the wood of *Prunus poddum*
   (a) *Vetiveria zianioides*, Poaceae
   (b) *Aruno donax*, Poaceae
   (c) *Cymbopogon citratus*, Poaceae
   (d) *Andropogon odoratus*, Poaceae

888. Seeds rich sources of the enzyme *urease*
   (a) *Dolichos biflorus*, Kulatha, Fabaceae
   (b) *Dolichos lablab*, sem, Fabaceae
   (c) *Vigna sinensis*, ramas, Fabaceae
   (d) *Phaseolus vulgaris*, bakla, Fabaceae

889. Which of the following is more effective in plant breeding
   work for inducing *polyploidy*
   (a) Superbine from *Gloriosa superba*
   (b) Clochicine from *Colchicum autunmale*
   (c) Colchicine from *Gloriosa superba*
   (d) Gloriosine from *Gloriosa superba*

890. Much used for making black ink
   (a) *Quercus infectoria*, mayaphal, fagaceae
   (b) *Canarium strictum*, black damar, Burseraceae
   (c) *Haematoxylon campechianum*, Leguminosae
   (d) *Acacia catechu*, Kattha, Leguminosae

891. Essential oil from seed is used as *Soap perfume*
   (a) *Anethum sowa*, dill, Umbelliferae
   (b) *Coriandrum sativum*, dhania, Umbelliferae

(c) *Foeniculum vulgare*, somf, Umbelliferae

(d) *Cuminum Cyminum*, Zira, Umbelliferae

892. *Jati (Jasminum grandiflorum, Oleaceae)* ghee is good for
   (a) Healing burns   (b) Stomach troubles
   (c) Edible purposes   (d) Eye troubles

893. Much used as *tonic for cattle*
   (a) *Euphorbia tirucalli* Euphorbiaceae
   (b) *Leptadenia reticulata*, Jivanti, Ascepiadaeae
   (c) *Pongamia pinnata*, Karanji, Fabaceae

894. *Banana sweet dessert* fruit is obtained from
   (a) *Musa paradisiaca*
   (b) *Musa paradisiaca var sapientum*
   (c) *Musa textilis*
   (d) All these

895. Pods and flowers are made into raita. Tender beans are eaten as vegetable.
   (a) *Parkinsonia aculeata*, Vilayati Kikar, Caesalpiniaceae
   (b) *Cassia occidentalis*, Kasundea, Caesalpiniaceae
   (c) *Bauhinia variegata*, Kachnar, Caesalpiniaceae
   (d) *Caesalpinia pulcherrima*, peacock flower, Caesalpiniaceae

896. Tree yields gum; bark tannin; Seeds yield fatty oil
   (a) *Poinciana regia*, gulmohar, Caesalpiniaceae
   (b) *Cassia fistula*, amaltas, Caesalpiniaceae
   (c) *Bauhinia variegata*, Kachnar, Caesalpiniaceae
   (d) *Saraca indica*, ashok, Caesalpiniaceae

897. It is considered as a valuable remedy in *asthma*
   (a) *Ruta graveolens*, rue, Rutaceae
   (b) *Zanthoxylum fraxinum*, Rutaceae
   (c) *Aegle marmelos, bael*, Rutaceae
   (d) *Myrica nagi, Katphal*, Myricaceae

898. Seasonal use as a prophylactic, deters the recurring of *malarial fever*
   (a) *Pilocarpus pinnatifolius*, Rutaceae
   (b) *Swertia chirata*, Gentianaceae
   (c) *Barosma betulina*, Rutaceae
   (d) *Clausena heptaphylla*, Rutaceae

899. Wood is important for *pencil manufacture*
  (a) *Juniperus communis*, Cupressaceae
  (b) *Tectona grandis*, Verbenaceae
  (c) *Gmelina arborea*, Verbenaceae
  (d) *Pinus wallichiana*, Pinaceae

900. Wood is used for making *walking sticks*
  (a) *Balanites aegyptiaca*, hingot, Simarubaceae
  (b) *Pongamia pinnata*, Karanji, Fabaceae
  (c) *Azadirachta indica*, neem, Mediaceae
  (d) *Polyalthia longifolia*, ashok, Annonaceae

901. Roots are rich in *diosgenin* which forms cortisone used for oral contraceptive
  (a) *Balanites aegyptiaca*, hingot, Simarubaceae
  (b) *Withania somnifera*, ashgand, Solanaceae
  (c) *Solanum nigraum*, gurkamai, Solanaceae
  (d) *Solanum nigrum*, gurkamai, Solanaceae

902. The fruit is used for cleaning *silk* and cotton
  (a) *Blanites azgyptiaca*, hingot, Simarubaceae
  (b) *Terminalia chebula*, harra, Combretaceae
  (c) *Terminalia catappa*, deshi badam, Combretacea
  (d) *Terminalia arjuna*, arjun Combretaceae

903. Excellent *brandy* and vinegar is made of the fruit
  (a) *Syzygium aromaticum*, clove, Myrtaceae
  (b) *Careya arborea*, Kumbli, Myrtaceae
  (c) *Barringtonia acutangula*, Myrtaceae, Samundar phal
  (d) *Syzygium cumini*, Jamum, Myrtaceae

904. Locally much used as a *hair tonic*
  (a) *Hemidesmus indicus*, Asclepiadaceae
  (b) *Hibiscus jatamansi*, Valerinaceae
  (c) *Nardostachys jatamansi*, Valerianaceae
  (d) *Impatiens balsamina*, Balsaminaceae

905. Seed is rich in Oil
  (a) *Phyllanthus emblica*, amla, Euphorbiaceae
  (b) *Phyllanthus niruri*, Zamin amla, Euphorbiaceae
  (c) *Croton bonplandianum*, Euphorbiaceae
  (d) *Baliospernum montanum*, danti, Euphorbiaceae

906. Word is used for *artificial limbs*, stethoscopes
    (a) *Avicennia officinalis*, Verbenaceae
    (b) *Verbenaa officinalis*, Verbenaceae
    (c) *Gmelina arborea*, Verbenaceae
    (d) *Petrea volubilis*, Verbenaceae

907. The bark of the tree is much sought after by arack manufac-
    turers to regulate the *fermentation* of toddy.
    (a) *Gmelina arborea*, Verbenaceae
    (b) *Avicei.nia officinalis*, Verbenaceae
    (c) *Lantana indica*, Verbenaceae
    (d) *Duranta plumieri*, Verbenaceae

908. *Gaozavan* of Indian bazars, used in bladder irregularities,
    blood - diseases, boils and eruptions, heart trouble (palpita-
    tion) etc. is obtained
    (a) *Onosma bracterafun*   (b) *Caccinia glauca*
    (c) *Priva laevis*   (d) *Congea tomentosa*

909. Which of the follwing are present in Caccinia glauca
    (a) Silica, lime   (b) Mangnesia, potash
    (c) Alumini with iron   (d) Carbonic acid, Soda

910. It is claimed that a necklace known as Kamla-ni-mala made
    of small pieces of the stem, has talismanic effection on
    jauundice.
    (a) *Tinospora cordifolia guduchi*, Menispermaceae
    (b) *Verbena officinalis*, Verbenaceae
    (c) *Callicarpa macrophylla*, Verbenaceae
    (d) *Lippia nodiflora*, Verbenaceae

911. What are the economic uses of *peel of banana fruit* (*Musa
    paradisiaca*, Musaceae)
    (a) The ash of banana peel is rich in potash
    (b) Dried peel is used for blackening leather
    (c) Ash is used in making soap
    (d) The peel is a useful source of pecting; peel and fruit
        contain anti fungal and antibacterial substances.

912. What are the economic uses of dye obtained from flowers of
    harsinghar (*Nyctanthes arbor-tristis*, Oleaceae)
    (a) Used as an auxiliiary to other dyes
    (b) Used for colouring liquors

(c) Used for dyeing wool
(d) Used for tanning leather

913. Match the following

(a) Root dye of *Onosma echinioides*	1. Dyeing wool red; for colouring pharmaceutical preparations
(b) Fibre of *Oreocnide integrifolia*	2. Ropes and sac cloth
(c) Pods of *Oroxylon indicum*	3. Dyeing and tanning
(d) Wood of *Ougeinia Oojeinensis*	4. Larger-beer casks and hogsheads

914. Match the following

(a) Wood of *Palaquium ellipticum*	1. Rubber chests, guide skids in mines
(b) Seed Oil of *Palaquium ellipticum*	2. Soap making; luminant
(c) Latex of *Palaquium ellipticum*	3. Adulterant of Heavea rubber
(d) Male flowers of *Pandanus tectorius*	4. Keora attar (perfume)

915. The burning plants serve as a *disinfectant* in a closed room and as an insect reppellent
(a) *Peganum harmala*, Rutaceae
(b) *Murraya Koenigii*, Rutaceae
(c) *Glycosmis pentaphylla*, Rutaceae
(d) *Fortunella japonica*, Rutaceae

916. Young leaves are cooked and eaten as *vegetable*. Forms an ingredient to 5 vegetables - Bauhinia malabarica, Amaranthus gangeticum Celosia and phalangium tuberosum
(a) *Cassia fistula*, Caesalpiniaceae
(b) *Cassia tora*, Caesalpiniaceae
(c) *Cassia sophera*, Caesalpiniaceae
(d) *Cassia occidentalis*, Caesalpiniaceae

917. Good for Soil reclamation
(a) *Adhatoda vasica*, Acanthaceae
(b) *Peristrophe bicalyculata*, Acanthaceae

208

(c) *Thunbergia grandiflora*, Acanthaceae
(d) *Andrographis paniculata*, Acanthaceae

918. Useful in *packing* or storing fruit and cereals
(a) *Adhatoda vasica*, Acanthaceae
(b) *Asteracantha longifolia*, Acanthaceae
(c) *Phlogacanthus tubiflorous*, Acanthaceae
(d) *Ruellia prostrata*, Acanthaceae

919. Leaves used as a green manure and also as a poison to kill the aquatic weed from rice field. Poisonous to any animalcules, frogs, leeches, fungi and insects
(a) *Adhatoda vasica*, Acanthaceae
(b) *Crossandra Sp.*, Acanthaceae
(c) *Barleria cristata*, Acanthaceae
(d) *Ecbolium viride*, Acanthaceae

920. Much used for seasoning nan bread
(a) *Coriandrum sativum*, Dhania, Umbelliferae
(b) *Trachysperum ammi*, Ajwain, Umbelliferae
(c) *Paucedanum graveolens*, sowa, Umbelliferae
(d) *Cuminum cyminum*, safed jira, Umbelliferae

921. What is the content of thymol in ajwani seeds
(a) 45-55 per cent   (b) 30-40 per cent
(c) 20-30 per cent   (d) 10-20 per cent

922. Leaves laid over grain are said to *keep off insects*. Leaf smoke *repels mosquitos.*
(a) *Gmelina arborea*, gamari, Verbenaceae
(b) *Lippia nodiflora*, Verbenaceae
(c) *Lantana camara lantana*, Verbenaceae
(d) *Vitex negundo*, Nirgundi, Verbenaceae

923. Match the following:
(a) Wood pulp in paper making   1. *Picea smithiana*
(b) Birja resin   2. Exudes naturally from the bark of pine
(c) Bakhar birja resin   3. Tapped from the sapwood of Pine
(d) Dyeing of tassar silk and wool 4. Bark off pine

924. Match the following:
    (a) Match boexs, match sticks   1. *Picea smithiana*
        and pines
    (b) Bodies of violins, sports requisites 2. *Pinus roxburghi*
    (c) Turpentine and tar   3. *Pinus roburghii*
                                               and *P. wallichiana*
    (d) Dyeing and tanning   4. Beaf galls of
                                               Pistacia integerrima

925. Wood is useful for making drums, tomtoms and other
     similar *musical instruments*
    (a) *Plumeria rubra* forma *acuminata*, Apocynaceae
    (b) *Plumeria rubra* forma rubra, Apocynaceae
    (c) *Thevetia peruviana*, Pili Kanar, Apocynaceae
    (d) *Nerium indicum*, Kanar, Apocynaceae

926. The dried leaves and branches are commonly used to *Scent*
     shawls, linen and other textiles and for flavouring country
     spirit.
    (a) *Pogostemon heynenanus*, Labiatae
    (b) *Mentha viridis*, Labiatae
    (c) *Ocimum sanctum*, Labiatae
    (d) *Anisomeles indica*, Labiatae

927. *Patchouli* of commerce
    (a) Dried branches of *Pogostemon heyneanus*, Labiatae
    (b) Dried branches of *Mentha pierita*, Labiatae
    (c) Dried branches of *Ocimum basilicum*, Labiatae
    (d) Dired branches of *Thymus vulgaris*, Labiatae

928. Industrial uses of *Punica granatum*, anar, Punicaceae
    (a) The dried rind of the fruit yields a fast yellow fye which
        dyes cloth green (Kakrezi)
    (b) Rind is used for tanning and dyeing morocco leather,
        hair dyes
    (c) Balustine (flowers) contain a tan and a fleeting dye
    (d) Stem bark is used for tanning and dyeing morocco
        leather. Root bark is used for making jet black writing
        ink. Root yield dyes.

929. The leaves soaked in water are used as *fodder for goats*. Dried
     fruit is used as a coagulent in the making of Cheese?
    (a) *Randia dumetorum*, mainphal, Rubiaceae

(b) *Rhazya stricta, hisawarg,* Apocynaceae

(c) *Thevetia peruviana,* pili kanar, Apocynaceae

(d) *Nerium indicum, Kanar,* Apocynaceae

930. The fruit yields a natural wax which is useful for making *candles* and *Japanese lacquer* work.

(a) *Anacardium occidentale,* Kaju, Anacardiacea.

(b) *Semecarpus anacardium,* marking nut, Anacardiaceae

(c) *Rhus wallichii, akoria,* Anacardiaceae

(d) *Rhus succedanea, Kakra singhi,* Anacardiaceae

931. Industrial uses of *castor Oil* plant, *Ricinus communis,* Euphorbiaceae

(a) Seed Oil used in making candles, calico printing, technical wax, soaps, hair oils.

(b) In the manufacture of roghan (used in making wax cloth), Turkey red oil

(c) Turkey red oil used in dyeing and printing of cotton end wollen fabrics; a fixing agent for alizarine dyes; dressing agent for tanned hides and skins.

(d) Seeds contain lipase; oil cake is a valuable manure.

932. The leaves are used for *manuring rice* fields

(a) *Pongamia pinnata,* Fabaceae

(b) *Nerium indicum,* Apocynaceae

(c) *Thevetia peruviana,* Apocynaceae

(d) *Parthenium sp.,* Compositae

933. Wood used in *railway coaches, ship sloons, billiard tables,* counter tops in banks and other places

(a) *Mangifera indica,* Mango, Anacardiaceae

(b) *Thuja occidentalis,* thuja, Gymmosperm

(c) *Dalbergia nigra, Brazilian* rose wood, Leguminosae

(d) *Pterocarpus indicus, Padauk,* Leguminosae

934. Economic uses of red gum, Kino, obtained from the bark of *Pterocarpus marsupium* gum Kinno tree Leguminosae

(a) Used in medical preparations

(b) Manufacture of some wines

(c) It contains 75 per cent tannic acid

(d) All these

935. What are the economic uses of *Pterocarpus santalinus,
raktachandan,* Leguminosae
    (a) Wood yields santalin dye used in calico printing, for
staining wood, dyeing leather red and cloth salmon
pink.
    (b) Wood is an ingredient of French polish, in Europe
    (c) Wood is much used as febrifuge and as a thirst remover
    (d) Wood is externally applied for inflammation, headache
in bilious affections and skin diseases

936. The leaves are used for *packing tobacco.*
    (a) *Pterospermum acerifolium,* Sterculiaceae
    (b) *Sterculia foetida,* Sterculiaceae
    (c) *Kleinhovia hospita,* Sterculiaceae
    (d) *Guazuma ulmifolia,* Sterculiaceae

937. As a well-known *rejuvinator,* the leaf-bud made into jam and
taken with milk for a fotnight
    (a) *Ficus benghalensis,* bargad, Moraceae
    (b) *Ficus religiosa,* pipal, Moraceae
    (c) *Ficus glomerata,* gular, Moraceae
    (d) *Ficus elastica,* Moraceae

938. Much used in the preparation of *silver*
    (a) *Urginiea indica,* banpalandu, Liliaceae
    (b) *Allium cepa,* Onion, Liliaceae
    (c) *Gloriosa superba,* glirlily, Liliaceae
    (d) *Asparagus racemosus,* Satawar, Liliaceae

939. *Gold* is present in the stem of
    (a) *Equisetum sp.*   (b) *Plagiogyria ferm*
    (c) *Selaginella Sp.*   (d) *Lycopodium sp.*

940. Young shoot lethal to *mosquito larvae*
    (a) Bamboo   (b) Bargad
    (c) Pipal   (d) Neem

941. The shoot extract shows *antibiotic* activity against *Staphylo-
coccus aureus and Escherichia coli.*
    (a) *Tridax procumbens,* Compositae
    (b) *Eclipta alba,* Compositae
    (c) *Parthenium argentatum,* Compositae
    (d) *Ageratum conyzoides,* Compositae

942. *Manjit dye* is obtained from which part of *Rubia cordifolia*, Rubiaceae
    (a) Roots   (b) Stem bark
    (c) Leaves   (d) Fruits

943. The reed is used for making *paper pulp*. The grass is a *good fodder for buffaloes*
    (a) *Saccharum munja*   (b) *Saccharum spontaneum*
    (c) *Themeda gigantea*   (d) *Imperata cylindrica*

944. What are the economic uses of fruit of star-anise, *Illicium verum*, Magnoliaceae
    (a) It is used. as a condiment for flavouring curries, confectioneries and spirits and for pickliing
    (b) The fruit is chewed to sweeten the breath and to help digestion
    (c) It is useful in flatulence, spasmodic affection of the intestinal canal and dysentery
    (d) It is used as an adjunct to cought mixtures and as a corrective of taste; used in perfumery in the production of absinthel (spirit)

945. Which of the following are *True?*
    (a) Rhizome of sweet flag, *Acorus calamus, Araceae* is used in perfumery industry
    (b) The rhizome of sweet flag is an aromatic bitter tonic and carminative used in dyspepsia and chronic diarrhoea.
    (c) The rhizome of sweet flag is useful against bed-bugs, moths, lice etc.
    (d) The :hizome is used in the manufacture of liquors, essences and bitters

946. What are the effects of *heroin injections* on the human body
    (a) Yawning, perspiration, running nose, teary eyes
    (b) Increased pulse rate, respiratory rate and depth, restlessness nausea
    (c) Increased blood sugar, vomiting, diarrhoea etc.
    (d) Pupil dilation, goose bemps, tremoss, loss of appetite.

947. It has not yet been possible to isolate and identify the chemical principles responsible for flavour, in which of the following fruits?
    (a) Apple   (b) Peach
    (c) Black currants   (d) Strawberries

948. Some fruit flavours may be the result of a single chemical compound as in
    (a) Apple   (b) Peach
    (c) Apricot   (d) Strawberries

949. How many chemical compounds are involved in the flavour of apricot fruits
    (a) 1   (b) 2   (c) 5   (d) 10

950. *Amchur* used as a souring agent for curries, chutneys, soups etcis
    (a) The dried product prepared from mango flowers
    (b) The dried product prepared from ripe mango fruits
    (c) The juice of ripe mango fruits
    (d) The dried product prepared from unripe mango flesh

951. *Amchur* is rich in
    (a) Citric acid   (b) Tartaric acid
    (c) Fruit sugar   (d) Glucose

952. *Anardana* mostly used as a condiment for acidification of Chutneys and certain curries, comprises dried.
    (a) The dried seedds (without flesh) of pomegranate
    (b) The dired seeds (dried wish flesh) of pomegranate
    (c) The dired bark of pomegranate
    (d) The dried fruit rind of pomegranate

953. Match the following: (regarding the uses of *Shorea robusta*, *Sal*, Dipterocarpaceae)
    (a) Perfumes and incenses   1. Chua Oil
    (b) Adulterant of ghee   2. Sal butter
    (c) Type writer ribbon, carbon   3. Ral (dhooma)
        papers
    (d) Railway sleepers, railway   4. Sal wood turn tailes, boat building

954. Match the follwing
    (a) Substitute for petitgrain oil   1. *Skimmia Laureola*, nair, Rutaceae
    (b) Leaves as incense   2. *Skimmia laureola*, nair, Rutaceae
    (c) Karai gum   3. *Sterculia urens,* Katila, Sterculiaceae
    (d) Substitute for tragacanth   4. *Sterculia villosa,* usal, sterculiaceae

955. Which of the following plants have *edible seeds*
   (a) *Sterculia foetida, Sterculia, urens,* Sterculiaceae
   (b) *Terminalia catappa,* Combretaceae
   (c) *Trigonella foenum - graecum,.* Leguminosae
   (d) All these

956. Leaves which have been soaked in water are used as sand paper for *polishing wood, ivory and horn*
   (a) *Ficus carica,* angir, Moraceae
   (b) *Morus alba,* Shahtoot, Moraceae
   (c) *Morus nigra,* black mulberry, Moraceae
   (d) *Streblus asper,* rusa, Moraceae

957. The powdered seeds are used to *clear water* in wells
   (a) *Strychnos nux-vomica,* Kuchala, Loganiaceae
   (b) *Strychnos potatorum,* nirmali, Loganiceae
   (c) *Symplocos sumantia,* Lodh, Symplocaceae
   (d) *Streblus asper,* rusa, Moraceae

958. *Nux-vomica* seed dye gives which colour to cotton fabrics
   (a) Green   (b) Pink
   (c) Yellow   (d) Brown

959. Wood used for *Ship building,* hulls of wooden ships, fittings of *battleships,* masts, spars; pit props in coal mines, railway carriage and wagon construction, railway sleepers
   (a) Teak   (b) Red sandal wood
   (b) Rose wood   (d) Sal

960. Wood used for bodies of *pianos,* organs and *harmoniums,* Keys of Violins
   (a) Teak   (b) Red sandal wood
   (c) Rose wood   (d) Sal

961. Which of the following are True?
   (a) Arjun *Terminalia arjuna* bark tannin is used for making fine upper leather and excellent sole leather of shoes
   (b) Fruit of *Terminalia bellerica* is used for making inks, for dyeing cloth and leather
   (c) Silver grey wood (*Terminalia bialata*) is used for ship's internal fittings, white chuglam (*T-bialata*) is used for motor body work, mathematical instruments.

(d) Leaf galls of *Terminalia chebula* are used in dyeing, tanning and for making inks. Tannic acid is prepared from the ribbed fruits

962. Fruits of *Terminalia chebula*, without ribs (*bhonga hirda*) are
(a) Used in tanning
(b) Used in Dyeing
(c) Not used in tanning and dyeing
(d) They are used for making durable inks

963. The astringent *gum* exuding from the bark is used in the preparation of cosmetics and as an incense
(a) *Terminalia tomentosa*   (b) *Terminalia chebula*
(c) *Terminalia arjuna*   (d) *Terminalia belerica*

964. *Murva fibre* is extracted from which part of *Sansevieria roxburghiana*, manjinaru, Liliaceae
(a) Stem   (b) Leaves
(c) Fruits   (d) Root - Stock

965. The sapwood of *Santalum album*, Santalaceae is used as
(a) Fuel   (b) Perfumery
(c) Cosmetic prepations   (d) Incense

966. The heart wood of *Santalum album*, Santalaceae is used as
(a) Fuel   (b) Perfumery
(c) Cosmetic prepartions   (d) Incense

967. Which parts of *Sapindus trifoliatus*, ritha, Sapindaceae are used as substitutes for soap in washing silk and woolen fabrics and in cleaning jewellery?
(a) Fruits   (b) wood
(c) Leaves   (d) Root-bark

968. What are the industrial uses of *Kusum oil* (*Schlieichera oleosa*, Kosumba, Sapindaceae)
(a) The oil is of great value in the manufacture of soap
(b) It is the basis of Macassar hair oil
(c) The oil is used for cooking and as a luminant
(d) All these

969. What are the industrial uses of Juice of fruit rind of *Semecarpus anacardium*, bhilawan, Anacardiaceae?
(a) Semi-hard and soft rubber goods

(b) Lacquers, varnishes, exampels
(c) Semisynthetic tanning materials
(d) Insulating materials, moulding plastics

970. What are the industrial uses of *Jamun* tree *Syzygium cumini*, Jaman, Myratceae
(a) The tree is a host of tassar silk worms
(b) Spirituous liquor (wine) and vinegar are made from the fruits
(c) Seeds are useful as cattle feed
(d) Wood is used in making agricultural implements, boat building, masts of boats, rice moratars, house building Bak is used in tanning and dyeing

971. What are the industrial uses of genda flowers, *Tagetes erecta*, marigold, Compositae
(a) Flower dye alum gives dull green colour to cloth.
(b) Unleached tassar silk give brownish yellow shade wish the dye
(c) Bleached tassar silk becomes light bronish yellow when dyed with genda
(d) The dye is used for colouring butter and cheese

972. Match the following
(a) For sizing country made blankets   1. *Tamarind seed cement*
(b) Planted as awind-break and Sand binder   2. *Tamarix aphylla*
(c) Galls on flowers, used in tanning sheep and goat skins   3. *Tamarix aphylla and T. dioica*
(d) Persian wheels, beds   4. Wood of *T.aphylla and T.dioica*

973. Match the following.
(a) Misri lei manna   1. *Tamarix aphylla*
(b) Pictine jellose   2. Seeds *of tamarind*
(c) Skum (tannic acid galls)   3. *Tamarix troepil*
(d) Gazanbeen manna   4. *Tamarix troupil*

974. The glycorprotein *miracularin* has the property of eliminating sourness or acidity temporarily (about an hour). Sour lemons taste as sweet as oranges it eaten after chewing the berries (which contain miracularin) of
(a) *Garcinia mangostana*   (b) *Annona reticulata*
(c) *Annona squamosa*   (d) *Synsepalum dulcifolium*

975. In the lemon, *limonene* makes up 70 per cent of the oil and *citral*, 5 per cent. Which are responsible for the lemon flavour?
    (a) Limonene   (b) Citral
    (c) Both limonen and citral   (d) None of these

976. *Carragheen*, with its pungent flavour due to a high potassium iodide content, is used as a flavouring plant carragheen is obtained from
    (a) Fungi   (b) Bacteria   (c) Ferns   (d) Sea weeds

977. The characteristic flavour of several famous *French Cheeses*, such as Bried, Camembert and Roquefort is due to the fungus
    (a) *Amanita*   (b) *Trichoderma*
    (c) *Puccinia*   (d) *Penicillium*

978. The *Greek wine* known as retsina is flavoured
    (a) By adding corriander seed powder
    (b) With the resin from the pine casks it is stored in
    (c) With leaves of *Mentha piperitc*
    (d) With leaves of *Thymus vulgar s*

979. The flavouring originating from confier, which is used in the production of *gins*, for flavouring in *meats, stews, roasts and in sauerkrant*
    (a) Juniper berries   (b) Pine cones
    (c) Hops   (c) Capsicum

980. Bark of *angustura, Cusperia febrifuga* is used for
    (a) Flavouring foods   (b) Dyeing fabrics
    (c) Tanning leather   (d) Cleaning metals

981. Leaf of *chives, Allium schoenoprasum* is used for
    (a) Flavouring foods   (b) Extraction of fibre
    (c) Extraction of Oil   (d) Extraction of rubber

982. Calyx of *roselle, Hibiscus sabdariffa* is used for
    (a) Flavouring goods   (b) Extraction of fibre
    (c) Extraction of dyes   (d) Exraction of tannius

983. Leaf of rue, *Ruta graveolens* is used for
    (a) Flavouring goods   (b) Extraction of dyes
    (c) Extraction of tannins   (d) Extraction of fibre

984. Which part of *balm* (lemon balm) *Mellissa officinalis* is used for flavouring?
    (a) Leaf   (b) Seed   (c) Bark   (d) Root

985. A spice which is exclusively produced in the new World
    (a) *Capsicum*   (b) Black pepper
    (c) *Pimenta*   .   (d) All spice

986. What are the economic uses of dried leaves of *rosemary*
    Rosmarinus officinalis, Labiatae
    (a) Added to cooked meats, fish, poultry
    (b) Added to soups, stews, sauces, dressings
    (c) Mixed with sage in pork and veal stuffing, sausages
    (d) Added to biscuits

987. Match the following
    (a) Sour cherry   1. *Prunus avium*
    (b) Sweet cherry   2. *Prunus cerasus*
    (c) European wild strawberry   3. *Fragaria vesca*
    (d) Cultivated strawberry   4. *Fragaria chiloensis*

988. Which of the following fruits is extremely *acidic*
    (a) Blackberries   (b) Strawberries
    (c) Blueberries   (d) Loganberries

989. They are one of the most perishable of crops and are usually
    not moved far to market
    (a) Banana   (b) Coconut
    (c) Strawberry   (d) Citrus

990. This diagram is the median longitudinal section of which of
    the following fruits

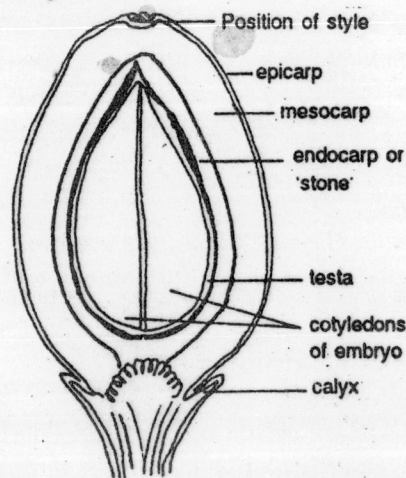

    (a) Banana   (b) Litchi
    (c) Strawberry   (d) Cherry

991. The plant breeding parameters and selection criteria for crop plants would be oriented for
    (a) Productivity per day, stable performance
    (b) Solar energy utilization, photoinsensitivity
    (c) Suitability for mechanical harvesting and processing
    (d) Quality of protein, amino acid profile

992. The opaque -2 hybrids and composites of maize have
    (a) Higher conten of lysine
    (b) Higher content of tryptophan
    (c) Higher content of water and salt soluble proteins
    (d) All these

993. The stalks and leaves of *Marsilia, Dryopteris, Pteris* are used as haerbage vegetables. The starchy paste of Sporocarps of *Marsilea drummondii* is prepared into cakes, called nardoo in Australia. These plants are
    (a) Algae   (b) Fungi
    (c) Bryophyta   (d) Pteridophyta

994. Match the following, regarding uses of *Pteridophytes*
    (a) Rhizome of *Dryopteris*   1. Medicines
    (b) *Equisetum debile*   2. To cure gonorrhoea
    (c) *Selaginella botryoides*   3. To cure liver diseases
    (d) *Lycopodium*   4. Stimulation for Kidney

995. *Silica* in therapeutically active form is found in
    (a) *Equisetum*   (b) *Dryopteris*
    (c) *Isoetes*   (d) *Lycopodium*

996. The ashes of which of the following *Pteridophytes* are used to relieve acidity and dyspepsia
    (a) *Equisetum*   (b) *Dryopteris*
    (c) *Isoetes*   (d) *Lycopodium*

997. What is the use of *Equisetum arveuse* in Pharmacy:
    (a) To relieve acidity and dyspepsia
    (b) To promote discharge of urine
    (c) To relieve gonorrhoea
    (d) Silica has haemostatic and haemopoietic properties

998. Which of the following *yield oil* (contains 50 per cent fixed oil)
    (a) Spores of *Lycopodium*

(b) Cones of *Selaginella*

(c) Spores of ferm

(d) Cones of *Equisetum*

999. *Kale, Swede, cress, water cress* belong to the family
- (a) Capparidaceae
- (b) Fabaceae
- (c) Papaveraceae
- (d) Cruciferae

1000. Which part of *Kale, Brassica oleracea var acephala* is used as vegetables
- (a) Stem tuber
- (b) Terminal bud
- (c) Leaves
- (d) Floral tissue

1001. Match the following:*Name of plant Part used*
- (a) Marrow stem Kale
- 1. Stem
- (b) Chinese Kale
- 2. Leaves
- (c) Brussels sprouts
- 3. Auxillary buds
- (d) Sprouting broccoli
- 4. Floral tissue

1002. *Calabresse, Swedes and brussels sprouts* are grown mainly in
- (a) India
- (b) Australia
- (c) United States
- (d) Egypt

1003. Match the following: regarding algal foods
- (a) Suimono
- 1. Dried fish + several sea weeds
- (b) Mitsu Sea weeds,
- 2. fruits, sugars and dried Kidney beans
- (c) Dulse
- 3. *Rhodymenia*
- (d) Seatron
- 4. *Nereocystis*

1004. Match the following
- (a) Nori
- 1. *Porphyra tenera*
- (b) Green laver
- 2. *Spirogyra, Oedogonium*
- (c) Kompu
- 3. *Laminaria, Alaria*
- (d) Asakusanori
- 4. Algae of Rhodophyceae

1005. Which of the following herbs are used in the preparation of an ancient Indian herbal drug *Chyawanprash*
- (a) Jivak, Risvak
- (b) Kakoli, Kshirkakoli
- (c) Meda, Mahameda
- (d) Riddhi, Vriddhi

1006. A secret medicine, in poweder form is in demand as putra-da (son-giver), for those, who want a male child. This is mostly made of ripe-fruit powder of

(a) Neem, *Azadirachta indica*

(b) Bargad, *Ficus benghalensis*

(c) Pipal, *Ficus religiosa*

(d) Aswagol, *Plantago ovata*

1007. Which of the following parts of atasi, alsi, *Linum usitatissimum* are edible

(a) Flowers   (b) Seeds

(c) Leaves   (d) None

1008. One of the most important *drying oil* for paints and varnishes

(a) Afasi (alsi) seed oil   (b) Groundnut oil

(c) Maize oil   (d) Soyabeen oil

1009. A mixture of carion oil - lime water and alsi oil is useful in

(a) Burns and scalds   (b) Cought and cold

(c) Eye trouble   (d) Gonty and rheumata trouble

1010. Match the following

(a) Analgesic   1. Pain - relieving

(b) Carminative   2. Relieving flatulence

(c) Diuretic   3. Promoting and increasing the flow of urine

(d) Expectorant   4. Promoting the discharge of matter from the throat or lungs by coughing

1011. The vegetable plant bhendi, lady's finger (*Abelmoschus esculenta*) grows better when grown on

(a) Green leaf manure   (b) Cow dung manure

(c) Hay manure   (d) Seaweed manure

1012. In Rajasthan, cartloads of which *algal* mats are which algae are thrown out from Sambhar Lake which are used by farmers as a *good manure*

(a) *Anabaenopsis*   (b) *Spirulina*

(c) *Spirogyra*   (d) *Cladophora*

1013. Which of the following *algae* yield *iodine*

(a) *Laminaria digitata*   (b) *Ecklonia*

(c) *Easenia*   (d) Few species of *Fucus*

1014. Which of the following *alga* is used in the extraction of *petroleum*; as packing material for bromine; in sugar refineries; cement, dynamite, rubber, blotting paper, soaps *insulation of boilers, blast furnaces*
   (a) Desmids
   (b) Diatoms
   (c) Spirogyra mats
   (d) Mats of blue green algae

1015. In Japan *artificial wool* is prepared from which of the following algae
   (a) *Sargassum*
   (b) *Nostoc*
   (c) *Rivularia*
   (d) *Spirogyra*

1016. *Red alga(e)* occurring in Black Sea, used in Russia for the extraction of iodine
   (a) *Ascophyllum nodosum*
   (b) *Harveyella pachyderma*
   (c) *Gracilaria confervoids*
   (d) *Phyllophora nervosa*

1017. The minerals of ash of a *red alga Ascophyllum nodosnm* of Black Sea, used in the extraction of Iodine
   (a) Gold
   (b) Tungsten
   (c) Silver
   (d) Zinc, aluminium

1018. Marine *alga* which are good sources of *potash*.
   (a) *Macrocystis*
   (b) *Nereocystis*
   (c) *Alaria*
   (d) All these

1019. The extract of which of the following *licheus* is effective against Tubercle bacili
   (a) *Pettigera canina*
   (b) *Parmelia Sp.*
   (c) *Rhizocarpon Sp.*
   (d) *Ramulina reticulata*

1020. Which of the following *algae* destroy bacteria *pseudomonas* and *Mycobacterium* and are antiviral
   (a) *Spirogyra*
   (b) *Nostoc*
   (c) *Cladophora*
   (d) *Lyngbya*

1021. World supply of *iodine* comes from
   (a) Brown seaweeds in Japan, France, Norway and Java
   (b) From sea water
   (c) From nitrate mines in Chile
   (d) From rock salt mines

1022. Among *algae*, highest copper content is found in
   (a) *Sarconia furcellatum*

(b) *Acanthophora Spicifera*

(c) *Durvillea antarctica*

(d) *Macrocystis pyrifera*

1023. Marine *algae* which contain potash 30 per cent in their dry weight

(a) *Macrocystis*   (b) *Nereocystis*

(c) *Sargassum*   (d) *Fucus*

1024. What are the vitamins present in *rice bran*

(a) Thiamine   (b) Nicotinic acid

(c) Pantothinic acid   (d) Niacin

1025. What are the economic uses of *rice bran* wax obtained as a by-product in rice bran-oil extraction

(a) It is used in chocolate industry

(b) Coating for candy and lozenges

(c) Preparation of wax emulsions applied to fruits and vegetables

(d) Cosmetics like lipsticks •

1026. Heat an iron pan containing sand. Throw rice into the heated sand, stirr rapidly, then sieve the rice for separating it from sand?. which of the following is prepared by this method?

(a) Flaked rice (Chura)   (b) Parboiled rice
                                        (Sela chaval)

(c) Parched rice (murmura)   (d) Parched paddy (Kheel)

1027. The filamentous mould *Aspergillus oryzae* or the thermotolerant basidiomycete *Sporotrichum pulverulentum* have been cultivated on cereal flours (barley), brans etc.

(a) For improving the quality of starch

(b) For improving the amount of fat

(c) For improving the quality of protein

(d) For improving vitamins

1028. In India, barley malted milk foods and malt extract are produced by

(a) Hindustan Milk Food Manufactuerers, Nabha, Punjab

(b) Cadbury Fry India Ltd, Bombay; Alvitone Laboratories, Madras; Foods, Fats & Fertilizers, Madras; South India Research Institute, Vijayawada; Mysore Industrial Testing Lab, Bangalore

(c) Mohan Meakin Breweries, Lucknow, Ghaziabad

(d) Jagatjit Distilling & Allied Industries, Hamira, Punjab

1029. Match the following

(a) *Avena brevis*   1. 2n = 14

(b) *Avena abyssinica*   2. 4n = 28

(c) *Avena sativa*   3. 6n = 42

(d) *Avena byzantina*   4. 6n = 42

1030. *Floating rice* is cultivated in which parts of India (harvesting is done by boats)

(a) West Bengal   (b) Assam, Orissa

(c) Tamil Nadu, Kerala   (d) All these

1031. Which of the following species of *Pennisetum* are cultivated for grain

(a) *Pennisetum clandestinum*   (b) *Pennisetum pedicellatum*

(c) *Pennisetum purpureum*   (d) *Pennisetum villosum*

1032. Which of the following *millet* crop is mostly cultivated in Koraput (Orissa); Bhagalpur, Darbhanga, Gaya, Hazaribagh, Ranchi (Bihar); Anantapur, Chittoor, Nellore, Cuddapah, Visakhapatnam (A.P); Coimbatore, Chingleput, north and south Arcot (T.N)

(a) Foxtail millet   (b) Pearl millet

(c) Sorghum   (d) Finger millet

1033. Match the following:

(a) Rice bean   1. *Vigna umbellata*

(b) Moth bean   2. *Vigna aconitifolia*

(c) Black gram   3. *Vigna mungo*

(d) Green gram   4. *Vigna radiata*

1034. Match the following

(a) Horse gram   1. *Dolichos biflorus*

(b) Velvet bean   2. *Stizolobium deeringianum*

(c) Cluster bean   3. *Cyamopsis tetragonoioba*

(d) Indian bean   4. *Lablab purpureus*

1035. Match the following millets:

(a) Jungle rice   1. *Brachiaria ramosa*

(b) Hungry rice   2. *Ziznia aquatica*

    (c) Wild rice   3. *Digitaria iburua, D. exils*
    (d) Browntop millet   4. *Echinocloa colona*

1036. Botanical name of *Australian millet*
    (a) *Coix lachryma jobi*
    (b) *Echinocloa decompositum*
    (c) *Paspalum scrobiculatum*
    (d) *Setaria italica*

1037. Botanical name of *Japanese barnyard millet*
    (a) *Echinocloa colona*   (b) *Eleusine coracana*
    (c) *Eragrostis tef*   (d) *Echinocloa frumentacea*

1038. Which of the following species of *ragi, finger millet* are tetraploid
(2n=4x=36)
    (a) *Eleusine coracana*   (b) *Eleusine indica*
    (c) *Eleusine africana*   (d) *Eleusine flagellifera*

1039. *Teff (Eragrostis tef)* is the most important crop (cultivated for grain) in
    (a) Ethiopia   (b) Kenya
    (c) Australia   (d) South Africa

1040. *Bombara groundnut (Voandzeia subterranea*, Fabaceae) Earthnut, Madagascar groundnut is cultivated in
    (a) Senegal   (b) Togo
    (c) Zambia   (d) All these

1041. What is the duration of crop (days to maturity) *bombara groundnut*
    (a) 120 days   (b) 100 days
    (c) 75 days   (d) 160 days

1042. What is the duration of crop (days to maturity) of *groundnut, Arachis hypogaea*
    (a) 120-135 days   (b) 100 days
    (c) 75 days   (d) 160 days

1043. *Shea butter* used in foods, cosmetics, as a substitute for cocoa butter in confectionery is obtained from the seeds of
    (a) *Achras sapota*, Sapotaceae
    (b) *Mimusops elengi*, Sapotaceae

(c) *Bassia latifolia*, Sapotaceae

(d) *Butyospermum paradoxum*, Sapotaceae

1044. *Shea butter* tree occurs mostly in
(a) West Africa   (b) Northern Uganda
(c) Southern Sudan   (d) All these

1045. *Cocoa butter* is obtained from which part of *Theobroma cocoa,* Sterculiaceae
(a) Seeds   (b) Bark
(c) Fruit rind   (d) Leaves

1046. What is the fat content in *rice bran*
(a) 2 percent   (b) 10-15 per cent
(c) 20-30 percent   (d) All these

1047. In the rice grain, *bran* comprises
(a) The germ   b) The pericarp
(c) Aleurone layer   d) All these

1048. What are the economic uses of *rice bran?*
(a) When refined, rice bran oil is a good edible oil
(b) Rice bran oil is used in soap industry
(c) Bran is used as a cattle feed; bran wax is used in chocolate industry
(d) Oil is used in textile, leather, flexible film, enamels

1049. Match the following

(a) Indian dammar (Indian copal)   1. Oleoresin from the trunk of *Veteria Indica*

(b) The bark is used for controlling controlling fermentation in toddy   2. *Vateria indica*

(c) The root yields a red dye used for dyeing cotton fabrics and tassar silk   3. *Ventilago madraspatana*

(d) It is exclusively used in the manufacture of attars   4. *Vetiveria zizaniodes*

1050. With chay-root the bark gives a chocolate colour; this combination is specially used in Mysore, Bellary and other towns of south India for *dyeing* brown borders of *cotton textiles.*
(a) Bark of *Ventilago madraspatana*
(b) Bark of *Ficus religiosa*

(c) Bark of *Ficus bengalensis*

(d) Bark of *Psidium guajava*

1051. Bark is used in the manufacture of *arrak* and gur
    (a) *Ventilago madraspatana*   (b) *Vateria indica*
    (c) *Verbena officinalis*   (d) *Viola tricolor*

1052. Essential oil is extracted from which parts of *Viola odorata*
    (a) Leaves   (b) Flowers
    (c) Seeds   (d) Roots

1053. The branches and leaves are *insect repellent* and so are used for preserving stored grains against insect attacks
    (a) *Vitex negundo*   (b) *Vitex altissima*
    (c) *Viola tricolor*   (d) *Valeriana sp.*

1054. The orange yellow juice of the wood is used for *dyeing wool* deep brown
    (a) *Thespesia populnea*, parash jhand, Malvaceae
    (b) *Hibiscus mutabilis*, guliajaib, Malvaceae
    (c) *Hibiscus esculentus*, bhendi, Malvaceae
    (d) *Hibiscus sabdariffa*, patwa, Malvaceae

1055. The grass is valuable for making good quality, *packing* and *wrapping papers* and also cheap badami paper
    (a) *Cenchrus ciliaris*, Gramineae
    (b) *Themeda arundinacea*, Gremineae
    (c) *Eragrostis pilosa*, Gramineae
    (d) *Imperata cylindrica*, Gramineae

1056. An excellent wood for *matches and match boxes*
    (a) *Trewia nudiflora*, Euphorbiaceae
    (b) *Ricinus communis*, Euphorbiaceae
    (c) *Phyllanthus emblica*, Euphorbiaceae
    (d) *Jatropha curcas*, Euphorbiaceae

1057. Temporary boats, called *tinho*, are made out of this plant for crossing rivers in flood.
    (a) *Scindapsus officinalis*, poria bel, Araceae
    (b) *Philodendron* Sp. Araceae
    (c) *Typha elephantina*, elephant grass, Typhaceae
    (d) *Anthurium* Sp. Araceae

1058. What are the economic uses of *Piney tallow* (Malabar tallow, Vateria fat) obtained from the seeds of *Vateria indica*, Dipterocarpaceae
   (a) It is used as a luminant
   (b) In the manufacture of soaps and candles
   (c) In confectionery
   (d) All these

1059. The *gum* that exudes from the stem is used in Mewar and Harauti for protecting parts of fabrics which are not to be dyed during the process of dyeing
   (a) *Woodfordia fruticosa*, Lythraceae
   (b) *Wrightia tinctoria*, Apocynaceae
   (c) *Wrightia tomentosa*, Apocynaceae
   (d) *Odina wodier*, Anacardiaceae

1060. The dried flowers of *Woodfordia fruticosa* are rich (up to 20 per cent) in
   (a) Tannic acid   (b) Glucose
   (c) Sucrose   (d) Benzoic acid

1061. The red dye obtained by boiling the flowers in water with the roots of *al* is used for *dyeing silk* and *cotton fabrics* and *leather*
   (a) *Woodfordia fruticosa*, Lythraceae
   (b) *Wrightia tinctoria*, Apocynaceae
   (c) *Wrightia tomentosa*, Apocynaceae
   (d) *Jatropha curcas*, Euphorbiaceae

1062. It is a favourite timber for the construction of *sea-going craft*
   (a) *Xylia dolabriformis*, Leguminosae
   (b) *Aescynomene aspera*, Leguminosae
   (c) *Sesbania sesban*, Leguminosae
   (d) *Tephrosia purpurea*, Leguminosae

1063. The bark and fruits are used in the manufacture of blacking of *leather*
   (a) *Zizyphus xylocarpa*   (b) *Zizyphus jujuba*
   (c) *Rhamnus franqula*   (d) *Rhamnus infectoria*

1064. Match the following *fruit plants* to their respective families
   (a) Blue berry, *Vaccinium myrtilus*   1. Ericaceae
   (b) Chinese gooseberry, *Actinidia chinensis*   2. Actindidiaceae

(c) Guava, *Psidium guajava*   3. Myrtaceae
(d) Carambola, *Averrhoea carambola*   4. Oxdalidaceae

1065. Match the following *fruit plants* to their respective families
(a) European black currant   1. *Ribes nigraum*
(b) Red cherry currants   2. *Ribes sativum*
(c) Gooseberries   3. *Ribes uva-crispa*
(d) Blue berries   4. *Vaccinium anguistifolium*
                              V. *corymbosum*

1066. Which of the following are True?
(a) Cold temperate fruit plants require chilling in winter to stimulate normal growth and flowering in the following year
(b) Those fruit plants that require little chilling need a long growing season and are damaged by dormant season frosts
(c) Those fruit plants given under (b) are classed as warm temperate fruits
(d) Tropical bananas, pineapples to those for dates, citrus fruits, apples, raspberries, currants are perennial and are vegetatively propagated.

1067. Fresh *olives* (*Olea europaea*, Oleaceae) are extremely bitter beacause they contain a compound that must be broken down or altered to make olives palatable
(a) Oleuropein   (b) Alkali
(c) Sat   (d) Oleoresin

1068. *Tabasheer* or *Banslochan*, a siliceous material a reputed tonic in Oriental countries, is obtained from which part of the bamboo plant?
(a) Tender leaves   (b) Tender shoots
(c) Culms   (d) Seeds

1069. Giant *bamboo* (*Dendrocalamus giganteus*) the tallest of bamboos, grows to which height in a day (24 hours)
(a) 1 cm a day   (b) 2 cm a day
(c) 7 cm a day   (d) 35-40 cm a day

1070. *Golden bamboo*, which has beautiful yellow and green striped culms
(a) *Bambusa vulgaris*   (b) *Bambusa tulda*
(c) *Bambusa arundinaceae* (d) *Dendrocalamus*

1071. *Male bamboo, Dendrocalamus strictus* differs from other bamboos in that
    (a) The culms are braqnched   (b) The culms are hollow
    (c) The culms are solid
    (d) The bamboo has male flowers only

1072. *Nectar* yielding trees
    (a) Barna, *Crateaeva religiosa* (b) Soapnut, *Sapindus* Spp.
    (c) Tun, *Cedrela toona*   (d) Shisham, *Dalbergia sissoo*

1073. Which of the following is a germplasm center for rice
    (a) IRRI, Phillipines   (b) ICRISAT, Hyderabad
    (c) CIP, Peru   (d) CIMMYT, Mexico

1074. West African Development Associattion (WARDA) is a center for research on
    (a) Soyabeans   (b) Sorghum
    (c) Wheat   (d) Rice

1075. Which of the following are direct sources of organic compounds - terpenoids, alcohols, long-chain hydrocarbons?
    (a) *Euphobia lathyrus*, Euphorbiaceae
    (b) *Euphorbia hirta*, Euphorbiaceae
    (c) *Brickellia* Spp. Asteraceae

1076. The bark of *Cascara tree, Rhamnus purehiana*, a most impotant product produced in North America, is in large demand for
    (a) Laxative purposes   (b) Edible food
    (c) Dyeing   (d) Spice

1077. Match the following fruits
    (a) Cherimoya   1. *Annona cherimoya*
    (b) Custard apple   2. *Annona reticulata*
    (c) Soursop   3. *Annona muricata*
    (d) Sweetsop   4. *Annona squamosa*

1078. *Hibiscus rosa-sinensis, gular* (Malvaceae) is called shoe flower beacuse
    (a) The inflorescence is shoe shaped
    (b) The flowers are shoe shaped
    (c) The staminal column is shoe shaped
    (d) The flowers are used to blacken shoes

1079. International Potato Center (CIP) is located at
    (a) El Batan, Mexico   (b) Uma, Peru
    (c) Ibadan, Nigeria   (d) Monrovia, Liberia

1080. CIMMYT (International Center for the improvement of Maize and Wheat) is located at
    (a) El Batan, Mexico   (b) Palmiro, Colombia
    (c) Rome, Italy   (d) Hyderabad, India

1081. International Center for Tropical Agriculture (CIAT) is located at Palmiro, Colombia is a germplasm center for
    (a) Wheat, triticale, barley and maize
    (b) Sorghum, pearl millet, pigeon peas, chick peas and peanuts
    (c) Barley, wheat, and lentils
    (d) Cassava, common beans, maize and rice

1082. International Institute of Tropical Agriculture (IITA) is located at
    (a) Ibadan, Nigeria   (b) Lebanon
    (c) Los Banas, Phillipines   (d) Monrovia, Liberia

1083. Which of the following trees yield *nectar*?
    (a) Neem   (b) Karanj
    (c) Mahua   (d) Eucalyptus

1084. Which of the following are resistant high salt in Soil?
    (a) Neem, *Azadirachta indica*
    (b) Palas, *Butea frondosa*
    (c) Mahua, *Bassia latifolia*
    (d) Amla, *Phyllanthus emblica*

1085. Which of the following trees is resistant to high salt in soil?
    (a) Lady's finger, *Abelmoschus esculentus*
    (b) Bhendi, *Thespesia populnea*
    (c) Shoe flower, *Hibiscus rosa-sinensis*
    (d) Mustard, *Brassica campestris*

1086. Which of the following are trees for Swamp and marshy areas
    (a) *Eucalyptus rostrata*   (b) *Salix babylonica*
    (b) *Salix tetrasperma*   (d) *Tamarix* Spp.

1087. Plantain (Kela) grows in swamp and marshy areas because
    (a) They produce underground rhizome
    (b) They produce aerial breathing roots
    (c) The broad leaves have a high rate of transipiration
    (d) The plant is resistant to salt

1088. What are the economic uses of *mahogany wood (Swietenia mahogany,* Meliaceae)
    (a) Manufacture of gramophone, radio and television cabinets, sewing machine covers
    (b) Pianos, organs, machine covers, medicine cabinet, jewellery boxes
    (c) Printer's blocks, rubbers, slide rules
    (d) In ship building, used for cabin fittings, rails, gangway, ladders, motor crafts, yacht deck fittings, companion wings etc.

1089. Which of the following timbers are used for making *musical instruments*
    (a) *Santalum album,* Santalaceae
    (b) *Azadirachta indica,* Meliaceae
    (c) *Mitragyna parviflora,* Rubiaceae
    (d) *Gmelina arborea,* Verbenacee

1090. Which fo the following timbers are used for making *agricultural implements*
    (a) *Acacia,catechu, A. arabica,; Anogeissus latifolia, Cassia fistula, Chloroxylon swietenia*
    (b) *Dalbergia sissoo, Diospyros melanoxylon,* Ougeinia dalbergioides
    (c) *Prosopis spicigera, Pterocarpus marsupium, Quercus dilata*
    (d) *Schleichera deosa, Shorea robusta, Tectona grandis, Xylia xylocarpa, Ziziphus murictina*

1091. Which of the following members of Araceae does not produce tubers
    (a) *Amorphophallus campanulatus*   (b) *Colocasia esculenta*
    (c) *Alocasia macrorrhiza*   (d) *Pistia stratiotes*

1092. Which of the following members of Umbelliferae produce *edible tubers?*
    (a) *Carum bulbocastanum*   (b) *Peucedanum dhana*
    (c) *Angelica glauca*   (d) *Bupleurum falcatum*

1093. Which of the following members of Papilionaceae produce *tubers*
    (a) *Vigna capensis*   (b) *Moghania vestita, M.tuberosa*
    (c) *Pueraria tuberosa*   (d) *Eriosema chinense*

1094. Which of the following members of Araceae are consumed as scarcity or *famine foods*
    (a) *Pothos scandens*   (b) *Pistia stratiotes*

(c) *Caladium bicolor*   (d) *Typhonium bulbiferum*

1095. The succulent shoots of *Caralluma adscendens*, *C. fimbriata*(maked shingi) are eaten as vegetable, The shoots are pickled, shoots are eaten cooked. *Caralluma* belongs to
(a) Araceae   (b) Asclepiadaceae
(c) Cactaceae   (d) Compositae

1096. Which of the following members of *Zizyphus* have edible fruits?
(a) *Z. apetala, Z. funiculosa*   (b) *Z. incurva, Z, mauritiana*
(c) *Z. nummularia, Z. oenoplia* (d) *Z. rugosa, Z. vulgaris*

1097. Which of the following members of Compositae have edible seeds?
(a) *Cirsium lipskyi*   (b) *Parthenium hysterophorus*
(c) *Acanthospermum hispidum* (d) *Calendula officinalis*

1098. Which of the following members of Papilionaceae have edible seeds?
(a) *Erythrina variegata var. orientalis*
(b) *Mucuna gigantea, M. prurita, M.monosperma*
(c) *Vigna capensis, V. pilosa*
(d) *Cicer soongaricum*

1099. Chief centres of coffee cultivation
(a) Arabia, Brazil   (b) India, Sri Lanka, Jawa
(c) France, W. Indies   (d) Parts of Africa, Indonesia

1100. *Congo coffee* is obtained from
(a) *Coffea arabica*   (b) *Coffea robusta*
(c) *Coffea liberica*   (d) All these

1101. The ancient Egyptians, Greeks, Romans and other early cultivations used this imperial *blue dye* of Europe for many centuries and was used by the ancient Britons as a body paint.
(a) Woad, *Isatis tincotoria* (b) Indigo, *Indigofera anil*
(c) Madder, *Rubia tinctorum* (d) Saffron, *Crocus sativas*

1102. Bark of Sassafras albidum, Lauaceae is used as
(a) Spice   (b) To flavour tobacco
(c) To flavour medicines   (d) To flavour gums; perfumes
    and soaps

1103.

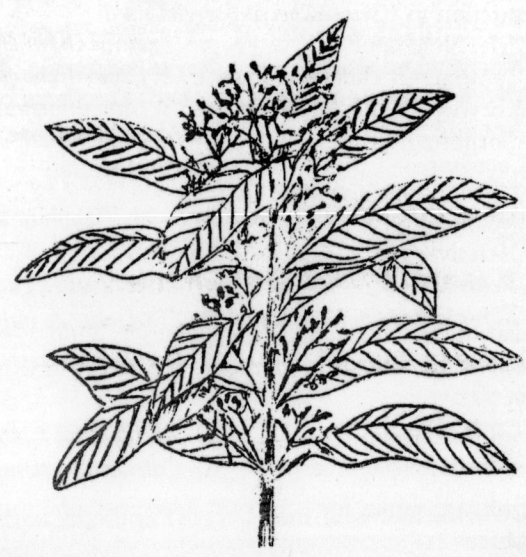

The plant given in the above picture is that of
(a) Cloves, *Syzygium aromatica*
(b) Black pepper, *Piper nigrum*
(c) Allspice, *Pimento officinalis*
(d) Cinnamon, *Cinnamomeem zeylaniceum*

1104. The wood yields a purplish -red dye and is used with iron salts in dyeing cotton, *woolen goods*, leather, furs and silk. It is used as a nuclear stain in biological techniques.
(a) Logwood, *Haematoxylon campechianum*, Caesalpiniaceae
(b) Cutch, *Acacia catechu*, Mimosaceae
(c) Sappanwood, *Caesalpinia sappan*, Caesalpiniaceae
(d) Red sandal wood, *Pterocarpus santalinus*, Fabaceae

1105. *Tea* of commerce is
(a) Dried petioles of leaves of *Camellia sinensis*, Theaceae
(b) Dried ripe mature leaves of *Camellia sinensis* Theaceeae
(c) Dried tips of leaves of *Camellia sinensis*, Theaceae
(d) Dried stems of *Camellia sinensis*, Theaceae

1106. Which of the following are drugs from roots and under-ground parts
(a) Ephedrine   (b) Santonin
(c) Asafoetida   (d) Nux vomica

1107. Match the following *cheeses* and the *fungi* used for flavor production in Cheese Cheese Fungus used
    (a) Brie, Nefchatel   1. *Penicillium camemberti*
    (b) Camembert cheese in France   2. *Penicillium caseicolum*
    (c) Norwagian skim milk cheese   3. *Mucor rasmussen*
    (d) Gorgonzola cheese   4. *(Penicillium gorgonzola*

1108. *Sufu* the chinese soyabean cheese is flavored by which of the following fungi?
    (a) *Actinomucor* Sp.   (b) *Mucor* Sp.
    (c) *Penicillum* Sp.   (d) *Aspergillus* Sp.

1109. Which of the following is the principal mold species in the manufacture of *Japanese Shoyee* (Soy sauce) and *miso* (Soybean paste)
    (a) *Aspergillus oryzae*   (b) *Actinomucor elegans*
    (c) *Rhizopus oligosporus*   (d) *Chlamydomucor oryzae*

1110. *Tempeh*, a popular food in Indonesia and adjoining areas, is produced by fermenting soybeans with the fungus
    (a) *Pencillium roqueforti*   (b) *Rhizopus oligosporus*
    (c) *Saccharermyces rouxii*   (d) *Aspergillus oryzae*

1111. *Ang-kak* or *red rice*, is primarily used in the Orient to color food,. It is an article of commerce in the Philippines, Indonesia, and China Ang-Kak is produced by fermenting rice with the fungus.
    (a) *Rhizopus oryzae* spores
    (b) *Penicillium camemberti* spores
    (c) *Aspergillus oryzae* spores
    (d) *Monascus purpureus* spores

1112. Which mold is used to tendrize and impart flavour to meat, usually beef
    (a) *Saccharonyces rouxii*   (b) *Aspergillus oryzae*
    (c) *Rhizopus oligosporus*   (d) *Thamnidium elegans*

1113. Fungi used in nucleotides, like monosodium gultamate (MSG) which is used in flavour enhancement in foods?
    (a) *Pencicillium citrinum*   (b) *Steptonuyces griseus*
    (c) *Aspergillus oryzae*   (d) All these

1114. *Ragi*, a fermentation product of Indonesia and China, is formed from rice flour which has been fermented by
    (a) Mold   (b) Yeast
    (b) Bacteria   (d) All these

1115. Match the following yeasts
   (a) Brewer's yeast   1. *Saccharmoyces cerevisae*
   (b) Wine yeast   2. *S. cerevisiae var ellipsiodeus*
   (c) Distiller's yeast   3. *Saccharomyces carlsbegensis*
   (d) Lactase production   4. *Saccharomyces fragillis*

1116. A yeast which lacks invertase, and therefore, can be used to remove glucose from egg material to effect color stabilization of the product during drying and storage.
   (a) *Saccharomyces cerevisiae*
   (b) *Schizosaccharomyces octosporus*
   (c) *Saccharmomyces fragilis*
   (d) *Candida monosa*

1117. Identify the following plant which is medicinally important in curing cancer.

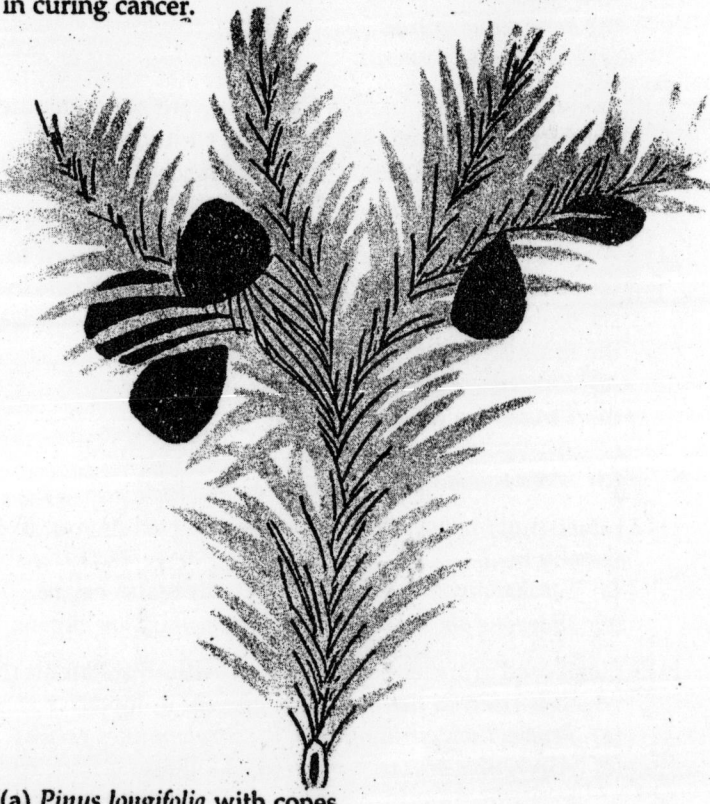

   (a) *Pinus longifolia* with cones
   (b) *P. sylveshis*
   (c) *Cycas circinalis*
   (d) *Taxus baccata* with seeds

1118. Which of the following plants are used as substitutes for *opium*
    (a) *Lactuca quercina*, Asteraceae used in France
    (b) *Mitragyna speciosa*, Rubiaceae; beaved used in Thailand
    (c) *Seeds of Pterygota alata*, Sterculiaceae, are used in Pakistan
    (d) *Lactuca viosa*, Asterceae; used in France; lactucarium is used in cough mixtures to replace opium

1119. The drug *heroin* is manufactured from
    (a) Opium obtained from *Papaver somniferum*, Papaveraceae
    (b) Ergot obtained from *Clavicaps purpurea* on rye
    (c) Mushroom *Psilocybe mexicana*, sacred mushroom
    (d) Leaf juice of *Cannabis sativa*

1120. *Dragon's blood* a dark-red resin is obtained the leaves and fruits of
    (a) *Draceaesa draco*   (b) *Daemonorops draco*
    (c) *Croton draco*   (d) All these plants

1121. Which of the following plants make a person " hot as a hare, blind as a bat, dry as abone, red as abeet, and mad as hen "
    (a) *Solanum tuberosum*, Solanaceae
    (b) *Solanum nigrum*, Solanceae
    (c) *Atropa belladonna*, Solanaceae
    (d) *Nicotiana tabacum*, Solanceae

1122. *Cinchona* bark is the world-wide remedy for which disease?
    (a) Typhoid   (b) Malaria
    (c) Vial hepatitis   (d) Flu

1123. Who was knighed in 1678 for curng Prince Charles II from malarial feVer with the medicine which consisted of Rose leaves - 6 drachms; Lemon juice - 202 and a strong infusion of Cinchona bark.
    (a) Robert Talbor   (b) Sydenhan
    (c) Joseph Pelietier   (d) Joseph Cacenton

1124. *Foxglove* is usefull in
    (a) Dropsy   (b) Fever
    (c) Diabetes   (d) Skin disease

1125. *"Kef"* in northern Africa and " *marijuana* " in the western world is obtained from
    (a) *Cannabis sativa*   (b) *Papaver somniferum*
    (c) *Erythroxylon coca*   (d) *Cola acuminata*

1126. South American *narcotic drinks ayahuásca*, ceapi or yaje
prepaed from the bark of a liana *Banisteriopsis caapi* or *B.
inbrians*, Malpighiaceae, leaves, leaves of *Psychotria* contain
   (a) LSD-25 (D-lysergic acid diethylamide)
   (b) DMT (N, N - dimethyl tryptamine)
   (c) B-carbalines (harmine, harmolive, tetrahydroharmine)
   (d) None of the above

1127. Plants used in South American *narcotic drinks* which give
hallucinogenic effect to the dinkers
   (a) Bark of *Banisteriopsis caapi, B. inebrians, B. rusbyana*
   (b) Leaves of *Psychotria catharginensis, P. virdis (Rubiaceae)*
   (c) Leaves of *Malouetia tamquarina, Tabernimontana
       (Apochsioides, Juanulloa ochraceae (Solanaceae)*
   (d) *Teliostachya lauceolata var crispa (Acanthaceae); Calathea
       veitchiana (Marantaceae), cacti, mints, sedges and ferms*

1128. The vine of *Banisteriospis* is cut into sections and allowed to
almost boil in a saucepan of water; the leaves of *Psychotria* are
added at this point and the two are simmered together for
about half an hour. The rust-brown liquid is cooled, then
bottled and corked. Which country prepared narcotic drink
in this way?
   (a) Brazil   (b) India
   (c) Japan   (d) Cuba

1129. *LSD - 25* the most powerful psychic drug known to man, is
how many times more powerful than mescaline?
   (a) 4   (b) 40
   (c) 400   (d) 4000

1130. Plants which contain *D-lyergic acid amide* and used by the
Aztecs and other Mexican Indians with divination.
   (a) Seeds of *Rivea corymbosa*
   (b) Seeds of morning glory, *Ipomoea violaceae*
   (c) *Tabernanthe iboya*
   (d) *Corynanthe yohimbe*

1131. *Ibogaine*, a comple indole alkaloid derives from tryptamine,
a hallucinogen, is obtained from
   (a) Dried root of *Tabernanthe iboga*, Apocynaceae
   (b) *Corynanthe hohimbe*

(c) *Alchornea floribunda*, Euphorbiaceae

(d) All these

1132. A red alga seawead used as carbohydrate source in making alcoholic beverages in *Kamchatka,* Siberia
  (a) *Harveylla pachyderma*   (b) *Polysiphonia fastigiata*
  (c) *Chondrus crispus*   (d) *Rhodymenia palmata*

1133. A fungus used as carbohydrate source in making *alcoholic* beverages in the tropics.
  (a) *Psilocybe mexicana*   (b) *Agaricus bisporus*
  (c) *Amanita muscaria*   (d) *Fomes auberianus*

1134. In Slavic countries, boilded leaves and fruit of which plant is used in making *alcoholic beverage*, bartsch.
  (a) *Zizyphys abyssinica*, Rhamnaceae
  (b) *Sclerocarya caffra*, Anacardiaceae
  (c) *Heracleum sphondylium*, Apiaceae
  (d) *Hyphaene crinata*, Arecaceae

1135. Which of the following are *opiate* lrugs
  (a) Morphine alkaloid
  (b) Heroin, formed by acetylation
  (c) Methadone, Synthetic
  (d) All these

1136. Which of the following are some of the 25 alkaloids obtained from *opium*?
  (a) Morphine 4-21 per cent
  (b) Codeine 0.8-2.5 per cent
  (c) Noscapine or Narcotine 4-8 per cent
  (d) Papaverine 0.5-2.5 per cent   Thebaine 0.5 0.5-2 per cent

1137. *Antibiotics* produced from *Streptomyces griseus*
  (a) Candicidin - B   (b) Cycloheximide
  (c) Steptomycin   (d) All these

1138. *Antibiotics* which has Gram +, Gram -bacteria and antihelmintic (kills helminth worms) activity
  (a) Hydromycin - B   (b) Ciprofloxin
  (c) Chloramphenicol   (d) Erythromycin

240

1139. *Antibiotics* acitve against Gram +, Gram- and tuberculosis bacteria
    (a) Paromomycin, Vancomycin
    (b) Knamycin, Viomycin
    (c) Neomycins, Streptomycing, Dihydrostreptomycin
    (d) Cycloserine, Rifomycin SV

1140. *Antibiotics* active against Gram+, Gram- bacteria and Rickettsiae
    (a) Chlortetracycline, Tetracycline
    (b) 6-Dimethyal-7- Chlortetracycline
    (c) Spiramycin, 5- hydroxy tetracyline
    (d) Chloramphenicol

1141. *Antibiotics* active against yeast and fungi
    (a) Nystatin   (b) Amphotericin B
    (c) Trichomycin, Variotin   (d) Candicidin B

1142. *Antibiotics* active against fungi
    (a) Griseofulvin   (b) Cycloheximide
    (c) Blasticidin S   (d) All these

1143. *Antibiotics* acitve against Spirochetes, *Treponema* which cause syphilis, yaws, pinta?
    (a) Penicillins   (b) Griseofulvin
    (c) Stendomycin   (d) Staphylomycin

1144. *Gibberellic acid,* cause of the " Backanae" or "foolish seedling" disease of rice plants and used as plant growth regulator is produced by the fungus
    (a) *Gibberella fujikuroi*
    (b) *Fusarium moniliforme,* imperfect stage of G. *fujikuroi*
    (c) *Fusarium oxysporum f- Sp- cubense*
    (d) *Fusarium udum*

1145. Which of the following are used to control *insect pests.*
    (a) Bacteria - *Bacillus papillae, B.thuringiensis; Coccobacillus acridiorum, Serratia marcescens*
    (b) Viruses-Nuclear polyhedrosis, Cytoplasmic polyhedrosis, Granulosis
    (c) Fungi-*Entompthora, Beauveria, Metarrhizium anisophliae* (Aeschersonia)

(d) Protoza-*Trelohania hyphantiae,Mattesia grandis Malameba locustiae*

1146. *Snuff* powder *hallucinogens* from plants
    (a) *Maquira sclerophylla* (*Olmedioperebea sclerophylla*), Moraceae
    (b) *Anadentanera peregrina* (*Piptadenia peregrina*), Fabaceae
    (c) *Justice pectoralis* var *stenophylla*, pulverized leaved added to Virola snuff.
    (d) *Virola calophylla, V. calophylloides, V. cuspidata, V. elongata, V. peruviana, V. Pumetata, V. rufula, V. sebifera, V. theidora,* Myristicaceae

1147. Reputedly sold in ports of southern Brazil as *substitute to marihuana*
    (a) *Cestrum laevigatum, C. parqui*, Solanaceae
    (b) *Atropa belladoma*, Solanaceae
    (c) *Mandragora officinarum*, Solanaceae
    (d) *Datura Sp.* Solanaceae

1148. Which plant is called ' *Leaf of God* ' and the leaf infusion of dried crushed leaves used as hallucinogen in Oaxaca, Mexico, by Chontal Indians (leaves also smoked)
    (a) *Iponoea violaceae*, Convolvulaceae
    (b) *Rivea corymbosa*, Convolvulaceae
    (c) *Salvia divinorum*, Lamiaceae
    (d) *Calea zacatechichi*, Asteraceae

1149. Fungus which is considered as significant tonic and stimulant for convalescents in China
    (a) *Codycepa sinensis*   (b) *Amanita caesaria*
    (c) *Volvariella volvaceae*   (d) *Agaricus campestris*

1150. Function of *folic acid* (Petroylglutanic acid), a vitamin of B-complex group.
    (a) CO_2 fixation, Carboxylation; Synthesis of fatty acids
    (b) Nucleoprotein synthesis; necessary in metosis
    (c) Coenzime in the oxidative decarboxylation of a-kets acids
    (d) Synthesis of protheombin

1151. Which of the following vitamin is important in the synthesis of prothrombin in liver for normal clotting of blood
    (a) K (Menadione)   (b) E (α-tocopherol)
    (c) D (calciferol)   (d) A, (retinol)

1152. *Wild ginger (Asarum canadense)*, root extract cures ear infections due to the presence of
    (a) Aristolochic acid   (b) Ibotenic acid
    (c) Psilocybin   (d) Muscimol

1153. For *hallucinogenic purposes*, experienced pickers have been eating the mushrooms
    (a) *Amanita muscaria*, fly agaric
    (b) *Psilocybe baecystis, P. cyanescens, P. pelliculosa, P. semilanceata, P. silvatica*
    (c) *Conocybe cynopus; Gymnopilus spectabilis*
    (d) *Panaeolus subbalteatus*

1154. *Mushrooms and fungi of hallucinogenic* use
    (a) *Amanita muscaria; Conocybe cyanopus, C. siliginoides*
    (b) *Gymnopilus spectalilis, Panaeolus sphinetrinus, P. subbaltatus*
    (c) *Psilocybe acutissima, P. hoogshagenii, P. isauri, P. mexicana P. mixaeensis, P. semeperviva, P. wassonii, P. yungensis, P. zapotecorum*
    (d) *Stropharia cubensis, Lycoperdon marginatum, L. mixtecorum (Puffballs); Claviceps purpurea (ergot)*

1155. Substance that stimulates mitosis and cell transformation
    (a) Mutagen   (b) Meiogen
    (c) Mitogen   (d) Mylagia

1156. *Mitogenic lectins* can stimulate B and T lymphoid cells to divide and mature. T cells respond to the phytoagglutinin (mitogenic lectin from plants that agglutinates erythrocytes and stimulates thymus-drived lymphocytes
    (a) Kidney bean, *Phaselous vulgaris*
    (b) Solubilized from of Concavalin A from the jack bean
    (c) Mitogen from lentil, *Lens culinaris*
    (d) Mitogen from *Wisterria floribunda*

1157. Drug or other orgent causing abnormal embryonic development in animals and humans, are called *teratogens*. Drugs which caused congenital malformations in humnan populations *(teratogens)* are
    (a) Thalidomide   (b) Aspirin, Cyclopamine
    (c) Corticosteroids, Cortisone   (d) LSD, Quinine

1158. *Antibiotics* which cause teratogenic effects
    (a) Actinonycin D, Chromomycin
    (b) Mitomycin C, Phlemycin, Streptomycin
    (c) Streptonigrin, Tetracycline
    (d) All these

1159. Fungal toxins / antibiotics which cause *teratogenic* effects
    (a) Aflatoxins   (b) Patulin
    (c) Penicillin   (d) LSD

1160. *Teratogens* from plants
    (a) Quinine from *Cinchona*, Cyclopamine from *Veratrum*
    (b) Cortisone from *Dioscorea*, mimosine from *Leucaena*
    (c) Sinigrin from mustard; ethyl alcohol; Sucrose from Suarcae, beet root
    (d) Caffeine, Nicotine, Mescaline, Colchicine

1161. Plants used for the cure of *asthma, cough and bronchits*
    (a) Small stem of *Vellozia equisetoides*, Velloziaceae, Twig of *Glyphaea brevis (Tiliaceae)*
    (b) Twig of *Napoleona leonensis, Lecythidaceae;* Roots of *Waltheria indica, Sterculiaceae*
    (c) Root of *Sphenocentrum jollyanum,* Menispermaceae; *(Phyllanthus engleri, Euphorbiaceae; Parinari curatellifolia,* Rosaceae
    (d) Root of *Mussaenda erythrophylla*, Rubiaceae; Root of *Cassia sieberiana*, Caesalpiniaceae Stem of *Clausena anisata*, Rutaceae; Twig and leaf of mango

1162. *Anti-sickle* cell factor is present in
    (a) Stem of *Fagara zanthoxyloides*, Rutaceae
    (b) Stem of *Murraya Koenigii*, Rutaceae
    (c) Stem of *Xanthoxylum rhetsa*, Rutaceae
    (d) Stem of *Ruta graveloeus*, Rutaceae

1163. Plants usefull in curing *ulcers, malignant tumors*
    (a) Stem of *Fagara zanthoxyloides*, Rutaceae
    (b) Stem of *Glycosmis pentaphylla*, Rutaceae
    (c) Twig of *Dialicum guineense*, Caesalpiniaceae;
    (d) Root of *Garcinia* kola, Clusiaceae

1164. When certain vegetable proteins known as *lectins* contact functional cell membrane glycorpoteins bearing polysaccharide side chains, they can combine to from bridges between cells, causing agglutination in vivo. They can induce killing of cancer cells and also as mitogens. Lectins are present in

(a) Balsam pear (Karela, bitter gourd), Castor

(b) Goundnut, jack bean (*Canavalia*), San hemp, Soybean

(c) Lentil, lina bean, Kidney been

(d) Pea, potato, common wheat, black walnut

1165. In Malaya, the deep-red heartwood of which plant is said to be used as a *remedy in heart attacks*

(a) Sausage tree, *Kigelia pinnata*, Bignoniaceae

(b) Mauve tabebuia, *Tabebuia speciosa*, Bignoniaceae

(c) Temple tree, *Plumeria acutifolia*, Apocynaceae

(d) Tulip tree, *Thespesia populnea*, Malvaceae

1166. *Rhododendron arboreum*, Ericaceae, whose florwers are acid in taste and are used for chutney-making by the hill people. The tree grown on

(a) Acidic soil   (b) Alkaline soil

(c) Soil with neutra pH   (d) Any type of Soil

1167. What are the economic uses of leaves of *Pongamia glabra*, Fabaceae, the pongam tree, *Karanj*.

(a) Leaves provide green manure in rice fields

(b) Leaves are used for cure of skin diseases

(c) Leaves drive away white ants

(d) Pongam oil from the twigs, is used in soap manufacture and skin dieseases

1168. Plants used in the cure of *leprosy*

(a) *Tamarindus indica* twigs; Root and stem of *Alchornea cordifolia* Euphorbiacea

(b) Stem of *Carpolobia alba and C. lytea* Polygalaceae

(c) Root of *Paulinia pinnata*, Sapindaceae

(d) Root and twig of *Piliostigma reticulatum, P. thonningii* Caesalpiniaceae; twig of *Acacia nilotica*, Mimosaceae

1169. *Teas* (leaves as a tea) used throughout the world

(a) *Ephedra trifurca* (Ephedraceae); *Artemisia abrotanum* (Asteraceae); *Lithospermum officinale* (Boraginaceae)

(b) *Viburnum cassinoides, V. theiferum* (Caprifoliaceae); *Catha edulis chat* (Celastraceae), *Celastrus paniculata* (Celastraceae); *Cyclopia ganistoides, C. subternata, Trigonella coerulea (Fabaceae)*

(c) *Chloranthus officinalis* (Chloranthaceae), *Cistus albidus* (Cistaceae); *Chamacedaphne calyculata* (Ericaceae); *Gaultheria procumberns* (Ericaceae); *Rubers caesiums, R. ideaus (Rosaceae)*

(d) *Croton argyratus, C. linearis,* (Euphorbiaceae). *Mallotus anamiticus, M. furetianus,* (Euphorbiaceae); *Frankenia portulacaefolia* (Fankaniaceae); *Malva sylvestris (Malvaceae); Epilobium angustifolium* (Ongraceae)

1170. Members of Lamiaceae leaves of which are used as *tea*

(a) *Cedronella triphylla, Clinopodium laevigatum; Glechoma hederacea,* gound ivy

(b) *Rosmarinus officinalis, rosemary; Satureja doreglassi,* Yerba buena

(c) *Sidertis thuzans; Stachys officinalis,* common betong; *Teucrium thea* used in China

(d) All these

1171. Members of Verbenaceae leaves of which are used as *tea*

(a) *Lippia citriodora,* Lemon verbena, *L. multiflora, Gambia tea bush; L. pseudothera*

(b) *Stachytarpheta jamaicnesis,* bastar vervain dried leaves for Brazilian tea

(c) *Verbena officinalis,* Vervain, dried leaves used as tea in Europe

(d) All these

1172. Match the following Plant drug Disease cure

(a). Taxol	(1) Anti Cancer
(b). Camptothecin	(2) Anti-cancer
(c). Castanospermine	(3) Anti-AIDS
(d). Hypericin	(4) Anti-AIDS

1173. Match the following

(a) Artimisinin	(1) Anti - malarial
(a) Tetra hydroxy indolizindine	(2) Cardio-toxic
(a) Camptothecin	(3) *Nothapodytes foetida*
(a) Forskolin	(4) *Castanospermum australe*

1174. Which of the following high value ornaments and foliage plants are in great demand and routinely grown on a commercial basis using tissue culture techniques?
    (a) Rose, carnation, gladioli, anthuriums
    (b) *Spathyphyllum, Diffenbachia, Cordyline*
    (c) Lilies, *Chrysanthemum, Gerbera, Ficus, Syngonium*
    (d) Orchids

1175. Match the following Plant Medicinal Compound
    (a). *Catharanthus roseus*   a) Amalicine
    (b). *Rauwolifia serpentine*   b) Amaline
    (c) *Digitalis lanata*   c) Digitoxin
    (d) *Artemisia annua*   d) Terpenoids

1176. A dwarf mutant rice TR-5, with non-lodging habit and condensed cigar shaped panicle was induce in the variety SR 263 using
    (a) Colchicine   (b) X-rays
    (c) Nitroso guidine   (d) Fast neutrons

1177. Rice variety *Hari* maturing in 135-140 days and yield of 6000 Kg/ hr, is obtained by
    (a) Crossing TR-5 with TR-8; and selection
    (b) Fast neutrons
    (c) Radiation treatment of De-Geo-woo-Gen
    (d) Crossing IR8 and TN 1

1178. Which of the following varieties of crop plants are obtained by using radiations
    (a) Black gram: TAU-1, TAUV-2, TAV-4; green gram TAP-7, TARM -2, TARM-1; pigeon pea: TT-6, TAT-10
    (b) Groundnut: TG-1, TG-17, TG-3, TGS-1, TAG-24, TG-22, TKG-19A,TG-26
    (c) Mustard: TM-2, TM-4; Jute: TKJ-40
    (d) Rice: Hari

1179. Match the following crop varieties
    (a) Mahadev TKJ-40   Jute
    (b) Trombay-Visakha TT-6,   Pigeon pea
    (c) Somnath TGS-1   Groundnut
    (d) Trombay- Akda-Tur 10 TAT-10   Pigeon pea

1180. The salt tolerant green manure plant *Sesbania rostrata* fixes 120-160 kg nitrogen / hecatre in 45-50 days. It has nitrogen fixing nodules on
 (a) Root   (b) Leaf
 (c) Stem   (d) Fruit

1181. The musical instrument *Violin* is manufactured from
 (a) Jack tree   (b) Sugar maple
 (c) Sisham   (d) Oak

1182. Match the following regarding the manufacture of *Violin*, a musical instrument
 (a) Bodies   1. Spruce and chirpine
 (b) Bridges   2. Jack and maple
 (c) Keys   3. Rosewood and ébony
 (d) Bows   4. Sundri

1183. Match the following regarding the manufacture of *Sitar*, a musical instrument
 (a) Body   1. Toon wood
 (b) Long neck   2. Teak wood
 (c) Keys   3. Sissoo
 (d) Bows   4. Sundri

1184. Match the following regarding *musical instruemnts woods*
 Musical instruments/ parts
 (a) Oak Wood   1. Organ bodies
 (b) Spruce Kail   2. Reed boards
 (c) Indian ash   3. Drums
   seris, sissoo and mulberry
 (d) Toon, halde, teak   4. Tom toms

1185. Which of the following woods is used in India in the manufacture of *guitars*
 (a) Indian ash   (b) Toon
 (c) White dhup   (d) Mulberry

1186. Which of the following are true?
 (a) Carnauba wax is obtained from *Copernicia cerifera*, Palmae
 (b) *Poeciloneuron indicum*, Ballagi
 (c) *Garcinia mangostana*, Mangosteen
 (d) *Calophyllum tomentosum*, Poor spar tree

1187. Foxtail millet, *Setaria italica* (Kangu) is cultivated mainly in
    (a) Andhra Pradesh   (b) Tamil Nadu
    (c) Assam   (c) Kashmir

1188. Bristly foxtail millet, *Setaria verticillata* (laptuna) is cultivated mainly in
    (a) Andhra Pradesh   (b) Assam
    (c) Gujarat   (c) Tamil Nadu

1189. Match the following:
    (a) Babassu oil   1. *Syagrus coronata*
    (b) Cohune oil   2. *Shorea aptera*
    (c) Licuri oil   3. *Orbignya cohune*
    (d) Borneo tallow   4. *Orbignya martiana*

1190. The poles of this tree are used for electrical transmission in Mysore.
    (a) *Mesua ferrea*, iron wood of Assam
    (b) *Poeciloneuron indicum*, Ballagi
    (c) *Garcinia mangostana*, mangostem
    (d) *Calophyllum tomentosum*, poor spar tree

1191. The ethyl ester of fatty acid of this oil is isolated and injected to *leprosy patients* for the relief
    (a) Colza oil obtained from the seeds of *Brassica campestris*
    (b) Argemone oil obtained from the seeds of *Argemone mexicana*
    (c) Sesame oil obtained from the seeds of *Sesanum indicum*
    (d) Chaulmoogra oil obtained from the Kernels of *Hydnocarpus kurzii*

1192. Which of the following leaves are used as *wi appers of tobacoo* in the bidi industry
    (a) Tendu, *Diospyros melanoxylon*
    (b) Apta, *Bauhinia racemosa*
    (c) Sal, *Shorea robuta*
    (d) Deshi badam, *Terminalia catappa*

1193. The wood of which tree is called *False sandal wood*?
    (a) *Santalum album*   (b) *Pterocarpus marsupium*
    (c) *Shorea robusta*   (d) *Semenia americana*

1194. Which of the following are soil enriching and *shelter belt trees*
    (a) *Gliricidia sepium, Tamarix aphylla*
    (b) *Corylus awellana*

(c) *Erythrina variegata var orientalis*
(d) *Acacia auriculiformis*

1195. Yellow (White wood) a soft light wood used in making musical instruments toys etc. is obtained from
    (a) *Michelia champaca*, Magnoliaceae
    (b) *Magnolia montana*, Magnoliaceae
    (c) *Talauna Sp*, Magnoliaceae
    (d) *Liriodendron tulipifera*, Magnoliaceae

1196. Guinea pepper, a spice os obtained from which part of *Xylopia aethiopica*, Annonaceae
    (a) Flowers   (b) Seeds
    (c) Leaves   (d) Fruits

1197. Highly *scented flowers* of Annonaceae
    (a) *Annona squamosa*, Custard apple, Sharifa
    (b) *Annona muricata*, Sour sop
    (c) *Canmaga odorata*, ylang ylang
    (d) *Artabotrys uncinatus*, Champa

1198. Seeds of *Nigella sativa*, alongi, Rannuculaceae are used as
    (a) Poison   (b) dye
    (c) Condiment   (d) Tannin

1199. *Medicinal* uses of *Ranunculaceae*
    (a) Stomach ailments   1. Rhizome of *Hydrastis canadensis*
    (b) Dropsy, jaundice splean trouble
        2. *Delphinium zalil*, asbar
    (c) Skin diseases   3. *Ranunculus falcatus*, baluchi
    (d) Febrill, inflammatory diseases
        4. *Aconitum napellus*, mitha zahar

1200. Match the following *ornamental plants* of Ranunculaceae
    Coomon name   Botanical name
    (a) Wind Flower   1. *Clematis*
    (b) Travelloor's joy   2. *Anemone*
    (c) Butter cup   3. *Ranunculus*
    (d) Butter cup   4. *Aquilegia*

1201. *Medicinal* uses of members of Nymphaeaceae
    (a) Dysentery   1. Tubers of *Nymphaea nouchali*
    (b) Heart diseases   2. Flower decotion of *Nymphaea stellata*
    (c) Diarrhoea, chloera   3. Flowers of *Nelumbo nucifera*
    (d) Liver troubles   4. Flowers of *Nelumbo nucifera*

1202. Leaves of *Crataeva roxburghii*, Capparidaceae are used as
    (a) Fodder   (b) Tannin
    (d) Dye   (d) Vegetable

1203. Match the following regarding *medicinal* uses of Brassicaceae
    (a) Asthma   1. Sees of *Nasturitium* indicum
    (b) Liver complaints   2. Leaves of *Lepidium Sativum*
    (c) Gonorrhea   3. *Labularia (Alyssum)*
    (d) Spices in food   4. *Melanosinapis, Sinapis* seeds

1204. *Medicinal* uses of Violaceae
    (a) Flowers boiled in water, used as   1. *Viola odorata*, banafshar poulitice in inflammalory affections of thorat, other parts of body
    (b) Gonorrhoea, urinary affections   2. *Hybanthus enneaspermus* bowel complaints in Children Ratanpurus
    (c) Diuretic, demulcent, tonic   3. *Hybanthus enneaspermus*, ratanpurus
    (d) Purgative in bilious affections   4. *Viola odorata*, banafsha

1205. The ornamental plants *Dianthus chinensis* (China pink) *Dianthus caryophyllata* (Carnations), D-barbatus (Sweet willium) belong to the angiosperm family
    (a) Viloaceae   (b) Caryophyllaceae
    (c) Portulaceae   (d) Malvaceae

1206. *Edible fruits* of Violaceae
    (a) *Leonia glycycarpa*   (b) *Viola odorata*
    (c) *Hybanthus enneaspermus*   (d) *Viola tricolor*

1207. Identify the wood of *Shorea robusta* from a & b.

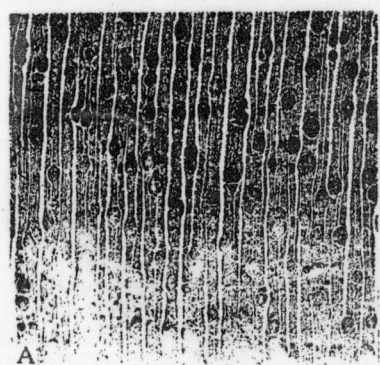
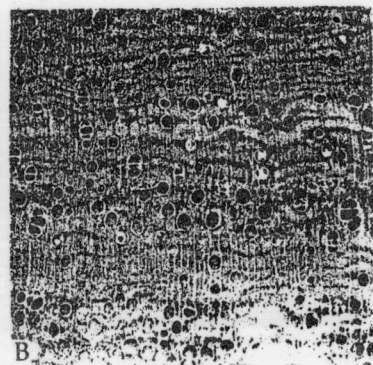

(a) *Shorea robusta*, sal; wood in tangential longitudinal section.

(b) *Dalbergia sisso*, shisham, wood in tangential longitudinal section.

1208. Identify the plant

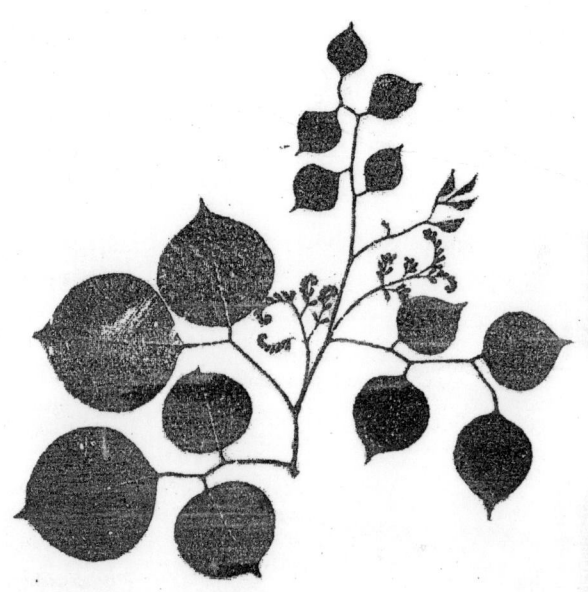

(a) *Dalbergia sissoo*, shisham
(b) *Pterocarpus marsupium*, red sandal wood
(c) *Dalbergia latifolia*, rose wood
(d) *Santalum albeum*, sandal wood.

1209. Economic uses of purslane, *Porfulaca oleracea*
(a) Used as green salad and cooked as vegetable
(b) Seeds are used as vermifuge
(c) Eaten by patients of effected liver
(d) *P. quadrifida* is bruised and applied in erysipelas; leaves are diuretic.

1210.

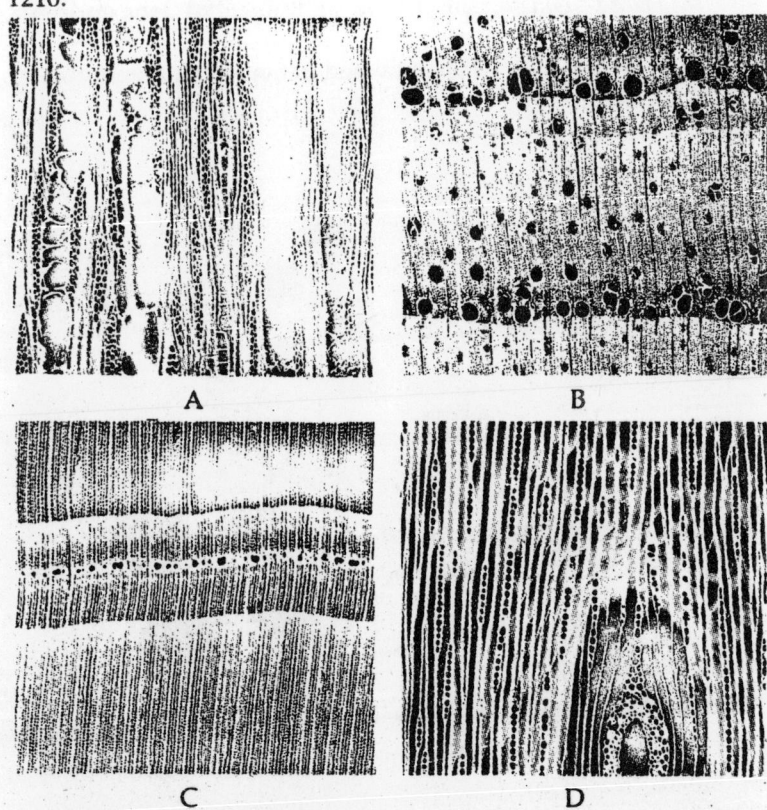

A

B

C

D

Identify above wood sections:
(a) *Tectona grandis*, wood tangential longitudinal section
(b) *Tectona grandis*, wood in transverse section
(c) *Cedrus deodara*, wood in transverse section
(d) *Cedrus deodara*, wood tangential longitudinal section

1211. Ornamental plants of Portulacaceae
(a) *Calandrinia, Anacampseros*
(b) *Ceraria, Claytonia, Calyptridium*
(c) *Levisia, Talinum, Talinipsis*
(d) All these

1212. Edible plant of Portulacaceae
(a) *Talinum*   (b) *Levisia*
(c) *Montia*   (d) *Calandrinia*

1213. Following the diagram of a member of Maliaceae

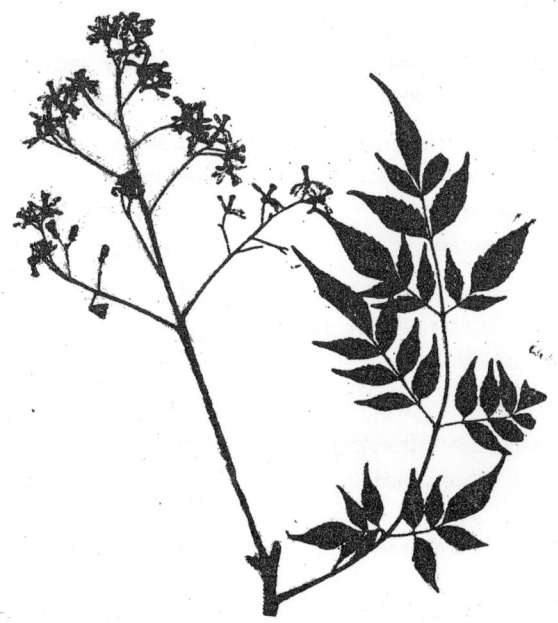

(a) *Azadirachta indica*   (b) *Swietania mabogani*
(c) *Melia azedarach*   (d) *Cedrela Toona*

1214. Following diagram is the wood section of

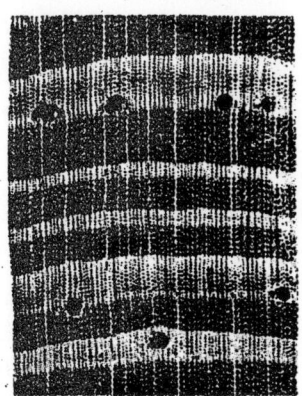

(a) *Dalbergia latifolia*, rose wood
(b) *Azadirachta indica*, neem

(c) *Swietenia mahogani*, Mahogany

(d) *Pinus roxburghii*, pine

1215. *Bimola oil* is obtained from

    (a) Neem seed   (b) Cotton seed

    (c) Mahua seed   (c) Sal seed

1216. Which part of *musk mallow* (*Abelmoschus moschatus*, Malvaceae) gives an essential oil used in perfumery

    (a) Seeds   (b) Flowers

    (c) Leaves   (d) Roots

1217. Which part of *Hibiscus rosa-sinensis* gurhal (Malvaceae) is used in *hair oils* for promoting growth of hair

    (a) Seeds   (b) Flowers

    (c) Leaves   (d) Roots

1218. Match the following

(a) Cotton plant	1. Root bark used for stopping haenorohage, after child birth
(b) Musk mallow	2. Roots used for the cure of stomach ache
(c) *Urena repanda*	3. Roots used as a cure for hydrophobia
(d) *Abutilon indicum*	4. Roots used against fever

1219. *French rose* oil or otto is obtained from which part of Pelargonium graveolens, Geraniaceae

    (a) Seeds   (b) Flowers

    (d) Leaves   (d) Roots

1220. *Geranium oil*, an essential oil is obtained from the leaves of

    (a) *Geranium ocellatum*, Geraniaceae

    (b) *Erodium Sp.*

    (c) *Pelargonium odoratissimum*, Geraniaceae

    (d) *Monsonia Sp.*

1221. Which of the following *tubers* are *edible*

    (a) Tubers of *Oxalis corniculata*, Oxalidceceae

    (b) Tubers of *Oxalis tuberosa*, Oxalidaceae

    (c) Tubers of *Oxalis deppei*, Oxalidaceae

    (d) All these

1222. *Folia taborandi*, leaves of *Pilocarpus pinnatifolius*, Rutaceae are

used for
- (a) Flavouring tobacco
- (b) Curing kidney troubles
- (c) Curing dysentery
- (d) Curing toothaches

1223. *Buchu,* a remedy for indigestion, is obtained from the leaves of
- (a) *Barosma betulina,* Rutaceae
- (b) *Clausena heptaphylla,* Rutaceae
- (c) *Luvunga scandens,* Rutaceae
- (d) *Evodia fraxinifolia,* Rutaceae

1224. Which of the fruits of following members of Rutaceae are edible
- (a) *Glycosmis pentaphylla,* bax ximbu
- (b) *Gortunella japonica,* Kumquat; F *margarita,* nagmi Keemquat
- (c) *Evodia fraxinifolia,* Kankpa, American bealch
- (d) *Clausena dentata,* Wampee: *C. excavata,* angijal; *C. lansium,* ampich

1225. *Japanese pepper* is obtained from
- (a) *Marraya koenigii,* Rutaceae
- (b) *Feronia oimonia,* Rutaceae
- (c) *Aegle marmelos,* Rutaceae
- (d) *Zanthoxylum Sp.* Rutaceae

1226. Match the following:
- (a) Leaves are used in
- (b) Leaves are used in
- (c) Leaves are used for
- (d) Leaves have the smell

1. *Aegle mearmelos bael, rutaceae*
2. *Clausena heptaphylla,* Rutaceae Flavouring tobacco
3. *Luvunga scandens,* Luvunga lata, worship in Hindu temples Rutaceae
4. *Murraya Koenigii mithanim,* Rutaceae

1227. *Jhingan gum* used in Calico-printing tanning and dyeing of silk is obtained from the bark of
- (a) *Odina wodier,* Anacardiaceae
- (b) *Semecarpus anacardium,* Anacardiacea
- (c) *Manogifera indica,* Anacardiaceae

(d) *Spondias pinnata,* Anacardiceae

1228. Match the following

    (a) Fodder for camels   1. *Alhagi camelorum,* Fabaceae

    (b) Used for folling rooms   2. *Alhagi camelorum,* Fabaceae insummer

    (c) Fodder for cattle   3. *Sesbania aegyptiaca,* Fabaceae

    (d) Fodder for elephants   4. *Butea monosperma,* Fabaceae

1229. Which of the following are *chewed with betel leaves* (pan) in India

    (a) Bark of *Derris elliptica,* Fabaceae

    (b) Bark of *Dalbergia tamarindifolia,* Fabaceae

    (c) Bark of *Butea monosperma,* Fabaceae

    (d) Bark of *Abrus precatorium,* Fabaceae

1230. Branch of this herb is kept under the bed or in any part of the house to control *bed-bugs*

    (a) *Abrus Precatorius,* Fabaceae

    (b) *Dalbergia sissoo,* Fabaceae

    (c) *Derris elliptica,* Fabaceae

    (d) *Desmodium pulchellum,* Fabaceae

1231. In which parts of India *mangosteen (Garcinia mangostana, Guttiferae),* " *Queen of tropical fruits* " is cultivated in

    (a) Kotttayam district of Kerala

    (b) Near Courtalam in Tamil Nadu

    (c) Lower slopes of the Vilgiris

    (d) Kallar and Buriar fruit station

1232. What is the extent of *mangosteen* cultivation in India

    (a) 2,500 acres   (b) 250 acres

    (c) 25 acres   (d) 25000 acres

1233. The only fruit in which glucose is in a readily available from for giving energy

    (a) Mango   (b) Mangosteen

    (c) Sapodilla   (d) Banana

1234. What are the economic uses of *mangosteen* fruit?

    (a) In Phillipines, an excellent preserve is made by boilding the edibloe flesh and seeds of mangosteen in brown sugar

    (b) The white translucent pulp is sweet and edible

    (c) Fruit contains 16.42 percent of total sugars and glucose in readily available form

    (d) The dried powder of fruit rind is a remedy for chronic diarrhoea

1235. What are the medicinal uses of *mangosteen* fruit?

    (a) Specific remedy for chronic diarrhoea and dysentery

    (b) The fruit is recommended for thrist in fever

    (c) The infusion of leaves is used in healing wounds

    (d) Root decoction is used for curing uterine disorders

1236. A cellulose - degrading fungus used in rapid *composting of straw*.

    (a) *Trichoderma harzianum*   (b) *Rhizopus stolonifer*

    (c) *Aspergillus niger*   (d) *Yeast*

1237. Much as for *fumigation*, in scent manufacturing and as a fixative

    (a) *Acorus calamus*, Araceae

    (b) *Abrus precatorius*, Fabaceae

    (c) *Achyranthes aspera* Amaranthaceae

    (d) *Aquilaria agallocha*, Thymelaceae

1238. *Liquor* fermented form fruit is good for indigestion, anaemia, Jaundice, certain heat complaints, cold in nose and for pranoting urination

    (a) *Emblica officinalis*, Euphorbiaceae

    (b) *Phyllanthus niruri*, Euphorbiaceae

    (c) *Ricinus communis*, Euphorbiaceae

    (d) *Euphorbia antiquorum*, Euphorbiaceae

1239. Used for making *baby's tonic, Gripe-water* specific for baby's stomach troubles

    (a) *Corcilum leptopus*, Polygonaceae

    (b) *Fagopyrum esculentum*, Polygonaceae

    (c) *Rheum emodi*, Polygonaceae

    (d) *Muehlenbeckia platyclada*, Polygonaceae

1240. Match the following

    (a) Root bark usefull in cancer of throat   1. *Viola odorata*

    (b) For curing haemorrhidd and prurigo   2. *Plumbago zeylanica* Piles, Ulcers

    (c) For curing ulceration of   3. *Berberis aristata*

pustular form
(d) For hastening suppuration,   4. *Cassia tora*
tumours and ulcers

1241. The galls produced by gall midge *Oligotrophys* on this plant, is used medicinally in the treatment of *whoopin ough*?
(a) *Juniperus*   (b) *Pinus*
(c) *Quercus*   (d) *Zizyphus*

1242. Which of the following are *Endangered orchids*?
(a) *Dendrobium amplum, D. chrysanthum, D. crystalinum, D. cretaceum*
(b) *Bulbophyllum, Habenaria*
(c) *Cypripedium cordigerum, Cymbidium eburneum*
(d) *Aconitum Kashmiricnum, Rauwolfia serpentina*

1243. Used for eradication of *Intestinal worms*
(a) *Centella asiatica*, Apiaceae
(b) *Sphaeranthus indicus*, Asterceae
(c) *Embelia ribes*, Myrsinaceae
(d) *Withania sonnifera*, Solanaceae

1244. This plant is used in combination with *Alpinia officinarum* for the treatment of *Jaundice*
(a) *Chrysanthemum coronarium*, guldaudi, Asteraceae
(b) *Eclipta alba, safed bhangra*, Asteraceae
(c) *Tagetes patula, genda*, Asteraceae
(d) *Sphaeranthus indicus, gorakhmundi*, Asteraceae

1245. This plant can improve *mental power*:
(a) *Eclipta alba*, safed bhangra, Asteracceae
(b) *Centella asiatica*, Bralami buti, Apiaceae
(c) *Tephrosia purpurea*, Jangli-nil, Fabaceae
(d) *Tagetes patula*, Genda, Asteraceae

1246. Crops cultivated by tribals for grain
(a) *Digitaria cruciata - esculenta variety*
(b) *Flemingia cestita*
(c) *Amaranthuus candatus*
(d) *Fagopyrum cymosum*

1247. Wild rice gathered and sold in the market in Orissa and in Rajahmundry (A.P)
 (a) *Oryza rufipogon*, wild rice
 (b) Seeds of *Bambusa arundinaceae*
 (c) *Coix lacryma-jobi*, wild rice
 (d) *Flemingia vestita*

1248. In West Indies, its branches are put into drinking water to make water cool.
 (a) *Mentha piperita*, podina, Labiatae
 (b) *Ocimum basilicum* (wild tulsi), Labiatae
 (c) *Ocimum sanctum*, tulsi, Labiatae
 (d) *Scoparia dulcis*, ghoda tulsi, Scrophulariaceae

1249. A cooling drink is prepared from the seeds by soaking the seeds overnight
 (a) *Scoparia dulcis*, Scrophulariaceae
 (b) *Russelia juncea*, Scrophulariaceae
 (c) *Antirrhinum majus*, Scrophulariaceae
 (d) *Veronica longifolia*, Scrophylariaceae

1250. Medicinal plants which cure leprosy and other skin diseases
 (a) *Aquiliaria agallocha, Cassia fistula, Centratherum, Anthelminicum*
 (b) *Caltropis gigantea, Psoralea corylifolia*
 (c) *Salix caprea, Semecarpus anacardium Terminalia beleriae*
 (d) *Cassia tora, Santalum album, Plumbago zeylanica*

1251. Plants which cure *ulcers and inflammations*
 (a) *Withania somnifera*, aswagandha
 (b) *Ficus religiosa*, aswatha
 (c) *Acacia nilotica*
 (d) All these

1252. A plant which cures skin diseases - *itches*
 (a) *Solanum indicum*, brihati
 (b) *Solanum ferox*, ram-begoon
 (c) *Solanum nigrum*, Gurkamai
 (d) *Solanum xanthocarpum*, Katita

1253. A excellent remedy for *Leucoderma*
 (a) *Psoralea corylifolia*, Bakeuchi, Fabaceae
 (b) *Ficus religiosa*, Pipal, Moraceae

(c) *Calotropis gigantea*, arka, Asclepiadaceae

(d) All these

1254. Which of the following is useful in veneral and *leprosy affections, scaly skin eruptions*
    (a) *Buchanania latifolia*, Anacardiaceae
    (b) *Semecarpus anacardium*, Anacardiaceae
    (c) *Odina, wodier*, Anacardiaceae
    (d) *Rhus parviflora*, Anacardiaceae

1255. *Diester*, a fuel in diesel engines which will burn as clearly as gasoline in cars with catalytic converters, is
    (a) Methyal ester of rape seed oil
    (b) Methyl ester of castor oil
    (c) Methyl ester of soyabean oil
    (d) Methyl ester of cotton seed oil

1256. Leaves improve *memory power* and can be used as " Brain Tonic"
    (a) *Poorana paniculata*, Convolvulaceae
    (b) *Evolvulus alsinoides*, Convolvulaceae
    (c) *Ipomoea purpurea*, Convolvulaceae
    (d) *Cuscuta anguina*, Convolvulaceae

1257. The plant is used with other combinations for the treatment of *Jaundice*
    (a) *Ipomoea reptants*, Convolvulaceae
    (b) *Evolvulus alsinodes*, Convolvulaceae
    (d) *Ipomoea bona-nox*, Convolvulaceae
    (d) *Ipomoea palmata*, Convolvulaceae

1258. *Salam gatta*, dried bulbons roots used as nutritive tonic are obtained from
    (a) *Vanda tesselata*, Orchidaceae
    (b) *Dendrobium nobile*, Orchidaceae
    (c) *Cypripendium elegans*, Orchidaceae
    (d) *Habenaria grandifloriformis*, Orchidaceae

1259. Members of Boraginaceae which yields a dye used to *colour wines, oils, pomades* etc.
    (a) *Heliotropium indicum*   (b) *Alkanna tinctoria*
    (c) *Trichodesma indicum*   (d) *Coldenia procumbens*

1260. Leaves are eaten in Northern part of Oudh as a *substitute for betel leaf.*
   (a) *Arnebia hispidissima,* Boraginaceae
   (b) *Cynoglossum procumbens,* Boraginaceeae
   (c) *Heliotropium indicum,* Boraginaceae
   (d) *Ehretia laevis,* Boraginaceae

1261. Match the following (regarding members of Mimosaceae)
   (a) Bark used in praparing spirits   1. *Acacia leucophloea* from sugar and palm juice
   (b) Heard wood yields kuch which is   2. *Accatechue*eaten with betel leaves
   (c) Bark is used as substitute for   3. *Acacia intsia* soap in washing hair
   (d) Leaves used as fodder   4. *Albizia lebbeck*

1262. Seeds after being roasted and powdered are used as a substitute of *coffee.*
   (a) *Caesalpinia pulcherrima,* peacock flower, Caesalpiniaceae
   (b) *Saraca indica,* ashok, Caesalpiniaceae
   (c) *Cassia occidentalis,* Kasunda, Caesalpiniaceae
   (d) *Poinciana regia, gulmohar,* Caesalpiniaceae

1263. Flowers are used as an excellent *uterine tonic*
   (a) *Bauhinia variegata,* Kachnar, Caesalpiniaceae
   (b) *Saraca indica,* ashok, Caesalpiniaceae
   (c) *Cassia fistula, amaltas,* Caesalpiniaceae

1264. Grown in newly plnated *Tea Gardens* as a fertilizer
   (a) *Alhagi camelogrum,* Fabaceae
   (b) *Dalbergia sissoo,* Fabaceae
   (c) *Tephrosia candida,* Fabaceae
   (d) *Derris robusta,* Fabaceae

1265. Which of the following members of Fabaceae yield *edible tubers?*
   (a) *Desmodium pulchellum*   (b) *Clitoria ternatea, apargita*
   (b) *Lathyrus macrorrhizus*   (d) *Pueraria tuberosa, bidarikand*

1266. Which of the following members of Mimosaceae are used as a substitute for soap
   (a) *Seeds of Prosopis spicigera*

    (b) *Seeds of Momosa pudica*
    (c) *Acacia farmesiana*
    (d) *Seeds of Entada pursaetha*

1267. Pods contain edible, sweet white pulp; seeds *contain oil*
    (a) *Pithecellobium dulce,* Momosaceae
    (b) *Albizia lebbeck,* Mimosaceae
    (c) *Xylia xylocarpa,* Mimosaceae
    (d) *Zamanea saman,* Mimosaceae

1268. Sweet pulp of the pods and bark are used as *famine food*
    (a) *Prosopis spicigera,* jhand, Mimosaceae
    (b) *Dichrostachys cinerea,* Mimosaceae
    (c) *Mimosa pudica,* lajwanti, Mimosaceae
    (d) *Acacia leucophloea,* safed kikar, Mimosaceae

1269. Gum from this plant is used for sizing paper in Nepal
    (a) *Albizia lebbeck*   (b) *Albizia stipulata*
    (c) *Albizia procera*   (d) All these

1270. *Shell* of the seeds is used in polishing boarders of the cloth called *dhotis.*
    (a) *Entada pursaetha*   (b) *Pithecellobium dulce*
    (c) *Albizia procera*   (d) *Prosopis spicigera*

1271. *Perfume* is obtained from the distillation of flowers of
    (a) *Acacia catechu*   (b) *Acacia suma*
    (c) *Acacia nilotica*   (d) *Acacia farnesiana*

1272. A member of Umbelliferae, which is a remedy for *leprosy* disease
    (a) *Foeniculum vulgare,* saunf, Umbelliferae
    (b) *Apium graveolens,* celery, Umbelliferae
    (c) *Coriandrum sativum,* dhania, Umbelliferae
    (d) *Centella asiatica brahni,* Umbelliferae

1273. Roots are used in the treatment of *annoeboic dysentery and dysentery*
    (a) *Rubia cordifolia,* manjit, Rubiaceae
    (b) *Anthocephalus indicus,* Kadam, Rubiaceae
    (c) *Cinchona calisaya,* Cinchona, Rubiaceae
    (d) *Cephalis ipecacuanha,* ipecac, Rubiaceae

1274. Match the following Dyes from Rubiaceae
    (a) Manjit (Yellow and red dyes) 1. *Rubia tincotira*
    (b) Fruit dyes   2. *Rubia tincotira*
    (c) Purpurin   3. *Randia uliginosa*
    (d) Alizarin   4. *Cordifolia*

1275. Members of Rubiaceae with *edible fruits*
    (a) *Anthocephalus indicus, Kadam*
    (b) *Vangueria madagascarensis*
    (c) *Cephalis ipecacuanha*
    (d) *Randia uliginosa*

1276. The insecticide *Pyrethrin* is got from the dried leaves of
    (a) *Wedelia calendulaceae,* Compositae
    (b) *Parthenium argentatum,* Compositae
    (c) *Tragopogon porifolium,* Compositae
    (d) *Chrysanthemum cinerariaefolium,* Compositae

1277. Fruits are eaten for cruing *rheumatism*
    (a) *Eugenia jambolana,* Jamun, Myrtaceae
    (b) *Rhodomyrtus Sp,* Goose berry, Myrtaceae
    (c) *Eugenia jambos,* gulab jamun, Myrtaceae
    (d) *Eugenia operculata,* raijaman, Myrtaceae

1278. Wood is very resistant to water effects and is used in *boat-making*
    (a) *Myrtus communis* common myrtle, Myrtaceae
    (b) *Psidium guajava* anmrud, Myrtaceae
    (c) *Barringtonia acutangula,* Samundarphal, Myrtaceae
    (d) *Eugenia jambolana,* Jamun, Myrtaceae

1279. Match the following:
    (a) Oil of Bay run   1. *Pimenta racemosa,* Myrtaceae
    (b) Jamaican pepper   2. *Pimenta dioica,* Myrtaceae
    (c) Cajaput oil   3. *Melaleuca Leucodendron,*
                                         Myrtaceae
    (d) Clove oil   4. *Eugenia caryophyllata,*
                                         Myrtaceae

1280. Fruits are used as a *remedy for dropsy.*
    (a) *Luffa cylindrica,* ghiatori, Cucurbitaceae
    (b) *Luffa acutangula,* Kali tori, Cucurbitaceae

    (c) *Lagenaria ciceraria*, Louki, ghia, Cucurbitaceae

    (d) *Luffa echinata*, Cucurbitaceae

1281. A cucurbit the leaves of which are *fed to silkworms*. Seeds are eaten after roasting

    (a) *Momordica balsamina*, mokha, Cucurbitaceae

    (b) *Melothria heterophylla*, Kundri, Cucurbitaceae

    (c) *Trichosanthes cusmerina*, rambel, Cucurbitaceae

    (d) *Hodgsonia hiteroclita*, tillau, Cucurbitaceae

1282. Compositae (Asteraceae) members with *edible roots*

    (a) *Chrysanthemum cineariaefoli*, Pyrethrum

    (b) *Tragpogon porrifolium*, oyster plant

    (c) *Helianthus tuberosus*, Jerusalem artichoke

    (d) *Helianthus annuus*, Sunflower

1283. Used *hair tonic*

    (a) *Wedelia calendulaceae*, Compositae

    (b) *Eclipta prostrata*, Compositae

    (c) *Tagetes erecta*, Compositae

    (d) *Calandula officinalis*, Compositae

1284. Members of Asclepiadaceae with *edible roots*

    (a) *Hemidesmus indicus*

    (b) *Pentatropis cyanchoides*

    (c) *Calotropis gigantea*

    (d) *Ceropegia bulbosa*

1285. Match the following (Medicinal uses of Asclepiadaceae)

    (a) Ulceration of mouth   1. *Oxystelma esculentum*

    (b) Janundice   2. Roots *of Oxystelma esculentum*

    (c) Boils   3. Leaves of *Marsdenia Volubilis*

    (d) Piles and gonorrhoea   4. Roots of *Asclepias curassavica*

1286. The roots yield aklaoid *reserpin*, which can lower blood pressure and tranquilize mental patients suffering from Schizophrenia

    (a) *Vinca rosea*, Apocynaceae

    (b) *Holarrhena antidysenterica*, Apocynaceae

    (c) *Rauwolfia serpentina*, Apocynaceae

    (d) *Carissa carandas*, Apocynaceae

1287. Which of the following are oil yielding grasses?
   (a) *Themeda gigantea*, Kapur ghas
   (b) *Imperata cylindrica*, dirhu ghas
   (c) *Cynodon dactylon*, Bermuda grass, doob
   (d) *Zoisia grass*, New Zealand grass

1288. Which of the following are oil yielding grasses?
   (a) *Andropogon odorattus*, ginger grass
   (b) *Cymbopogon citratus*, Lemon grass
   (c) *Cymbopogon martini*, gernium oil grass
   (d) *Cymbopogon nardus*, Citronella grass

1289. Which of the folloiwng are pseudocereals
   (a) Ragi, *Eleusine coracana*; Jiwar, *Sorghum vulgare*
   (b) Canada rice, *Zizania aquatica*; Buck wheat, Kutu, *Fagopyrum esculentum*, Polygonaceae
   (c) Rye, *Secale cerale*; Oat jaee, *Avena sativa*
   (d) Barley jow, *Howdeum vulgare*; pearl millet, bajra *Pennisetum glaucum* and *P. typhoideum*

1290. Nuts with high fat content
   (a) Pistachio nuts, Pista   (b) Almonds, badam
   (c) Beach nut, *Fagus Sp.*   (d) Wallnuts, Akhrot

1291. Nuts with high fat content
   (a) Chestnut, *Castanea Sp*
   (b) Acorns *Quercus Sp.*
   (c) Green almonds, *Pistacia Sp*
   (d) Pine nuts, Chilgoza

1292. Cashew nuts, Kaju, *Anacardium occidentale*
   (a) Nuts with high carbohydrate content
   (b) Nuts with high fat content
   (c) Nuts with high protein content
   (d) Nuts with high carbohydrate, high fat and high portein content

1293. Which of the following woods yield cork, cork is used as stoppers for bottles, hats, cigaette tips, insulating material in refrigeration; and in high speed jet plantes and in sound proof rooms
   (a) Cedar wood from *Cedrus deodara*, gymnosperm

(b) Wood of *Quercus suber*, Fagaceae

(c) Wood of *Mangifera indica*, Anacardiaceae

(d) Rose wood from *Dalbergia latifolia D. Sissoo*, Leguminosae

1294. Wood suitable for modeling *aircaft*
- (a) Balsa, *Ochroma lagopus*
- (b) Cork, *Quercus suber*
- (c) Wood of *Aeschynome aspera*
- (d) Thuja wood, *Thuja occidentalis*

1295. In India *hockey sticks* are generally made from the wood of
- (a) *Morus alba*
- (b) *Dalbergia latifolia*
- (c) *Mangifera indica*
- (d) *Cedrus deodara*

1296. In India cricket bats are generally made from
- (a) *Salix alba*, Willow
- (b) *Pinus wallichiana*, Pine
- (c) *Juniperus virginiana*, Juniper
- (d) *Cedrus deodara*, Deodar

1297. *Bottle cork* is obtained from
- (a) *Quercus suber*
- (b) *Aeschynomene aspera*
- (c) *Tectona grandis*
- (d) *Santalum album*

1298. *Rifle parts* are made from the wood of
- (a) *Swietenia* mahogany
- (b) *Quercus*, Oak
- (c) *Juglans* Sp. Walnut
- (d) *Salix* Sp. Willow

1299. Wood used in making *hockey sticks*, tennis and badminton rackets, cricket stumps etc.
- (a) *Morus alba*, mulberry
- (b) *Ficus benghalensis* bargad
- (c) *Mangifera indica*, Mango
- (d) *Eucalyptus Sp.*

1300. In philippines, the fruits of which of the following plant are used as *torch lights* (bamboo tubes are filled with fruits and ignited)
- (a) *Pittosporum resiniferum*
- (b) *Linum usitatissimum*
- (c) *Ricinus communis*
- (d) *Cocos nucifera*

ANSWERS

Note : E : All correct,   F : All Wrong

1.	a	39.	a,c	77.	d	115.	d
2.	a	40.	a,b	78.	d	116.	c
3.	a	41.	a,c	79.	e	117.	d
4.	a	42.	e	80.	a	118.	d
5.	a	43.	e	81.	a,b	119.	a
6.	e	44.	e	82.	a,b	120.	a
7.	e	45.	d	83.	e	121.	a
8.	d	46.	a	84.	e	122.	a
9.	d	47.	d	85.	a	123.	b
10.	c	48.	a	86.	a	124.	d
11.	e	49.	a	87.	e	125.	b
12.	a	50.	a	88.	e	126.	e
13.	e	51.	a	89.	e	127.	a,b
14.	d	52.	d	90.	a	128.	a
15.	e	53.	c	91.	a	129.	d
16.	a	54.	a	92.	d	130.	e
17.	a	55.	c	93.	d	131.	e
18.	c	56.	b	94.	b	132.	e
19.	d	57.	d	95.	a	133.	b
20.	b	58.	d	96.	e	134.	b
21.	c,d	59.	a	97.	a	135.	a
22.	a,b	60.	d	98.	e	136.	e
23.	a	61.	a	99.	e	137.	b
24.	a	62.	a	100.	a,b	138.	a,b
25.	a	63.	d	101.	d	139.	c
26.	a	64.	d	102.	b	140.	d
27.	a	65.	d	103.	e	141.	b
28.	a	66.	b	104.	d	142.	a
29.	b	67.	c	105.	d	143.	d
30.	a	68.	a	106.	a	144.	d
31.	a	69.	d	107.	d	145.	a
32.	a	70.	d	108.	b,c	146.	d
33.	b	71.	e	109.	b	147.	a
34.	a	72.	d	110.	c	148.	d
35.	c,d	73.	e	111.	e	149.	e
36.	b,c	74.	a	112.	a	150.	e
37.	c	75.	a,b	113.	d	151.	d
38.	a,b	76.	a	114.	e	152.	a

No.	Ans.	No.	Ans.	No.	Ans.	No.	Ans.
153.	a	195.	a	237.	c	279.	c
154.	c	196.	a	238.	a	280.	d
155.	a	197.	a	239.	c	281.	d
156.	d	198.	c	240.	d	282.	d
157.	c	199.	b	241.	a	283.	d
158.	d	200.	a	242.	c,d	284.	a
159.	a	201.	a	243.	d	285.	a
160.	c	202.	d	244.	a	286.	d
161.	d	203.	c	245.	d	287.	c
162.	c	204.	d	246.		288.	b
163.	d	205.	b	247.	a,c	289.	a
164.	b	206.	a	248.	e	290.	a
165.	c	207.	e	249.	b	291.	c,d
166.	d	208.	a,d	250.	c	292.	d
167.	c	209.	a	251.	c	293.	d
168.	d	210.	a,b	252.	a	294.	b
169.	b	211.	a,b	253.	b	295.	d
170.	d	212.	a	254.	a	296.	c
171.	d	213.	a,b	255.	d	297.	d
172.	a	214.	d	256.	d	298.	b
173.	a	215.	d	257.	a	299.	a
174.	a	216.	b	258.	a	300.	c
175.	a	217.	e	259.	a	301.	d
176.	d	218.	b	260.	a,c	302.	a
177.	a,b	219.	e	261.	a	303.	b
178.	b	220.	c	262.	a	304.	a
179.	e	221.	d	263.	c	305.	b
180.	d	222.	d	264.	b	306.	a
181.	a	223.	b	265.	e	307.	c
182.	d	224.	b	266.	d	308.	b
183.	e	225.	a	267.	a	309.	d
184.	d	226.	a	268.	c	310.	a
185.	d	227.	a	269.	d	311.	c,d
186.	d	228.	e	270.	b	312.	c
187.	e	229.	a	271.	a	313.	c
188.	d	230.	a,b	272.	b	314.	a
189.	b	231.	c	273.	e	315.	d
190.	b	232.	b	274.	d	316.	a
191.	b	233.	b	275.	a	317.	a
192.	d	234.	d	276.	b	318.	a
193.	a	235.	a	277.	c	319.	d
194.	b	236.	c	278.	c	320.	d

321.	c	363.	a	405.	d	447.	e
322.	c	364.	d	406.	e	448.	e
323.	a	365.	a	407.	e	449.	a,b
324.	d	366.	d	408.	d	450.	a
325.	e	367.	a	409.	d	451.	d
326.	e	368.	c	410.	a	452.	a
327.	a	369.	d	411.	e	453.	d
328.	e	370.	a	412.	e	454.	e
329.	c	371.	e	413.		455.	d
330.	c,d	372.	e	414.	d	456.	d
331.	d	373.	d	415.	d	457.	a
332.	d	374.	a	416.	d	458.	b
333.	d	375.	e	417.	e	459.	b
334.	d	376.	c	418.	c	460.	a
335.	a	377.	e	419.	a,b	461.	c
376.		378.	d	420.	e	462.	d
337.	a	379.	c	421.	b	463.	d
338.	a	380.	a	422.	d	464.	e
339.	a	381.	d	423.	a	465.	a
340.	d	382.	a	424.	b	466.	a
341.	a	383.	a	425.	b,c	467.	d
342.	e	384.	a	426.	d	468.	d
343.	d	385.	a	427.	a	469.	e
344.	b,c	386.	d	428.	d	470.	e
345.	a,b	387.	d	429.	a	471.	e
346.	b,c	388.	a	430.	e	472.	d
347.	a	389.	b	431.	e	473.	d
348.	b	390.	b	432.	a	474.	e
349.	a	391.	a	433.	e	475.	e
350.	a	392.	a	434.	e	476.	d
351.	e	393.	e	435.	a	477.	a,b
352.	d	394.	a	436.	c	478.	a
353.	c	395.	c	437.	e	479.	d
354.	a	396.	b	438.	c	480.	b
355.	a	397.	b	439.	d	481.	d
356.	d	398.	d	440.	a,c	482.	c
357.	b	399.	a,b	441.	a	483.	a,b
358.	c	400.	b	442.	a,b	484.	c
359.	a	401.	d	443.	e	485.	b
360.	a,b	402.	d	444.	e	486.	c
361.	c	403.	e	445.	c,d	487.	a
362.	e	404.	b	446.	e	488.	e

489. a	531. a	b-2	608. c
490. d	532. c	c-3	609. d
491. a,b	533. a	d-4	610. e
492. a	534. d	570. d	611. e
493. d	535. d	571. d	612. c
494. d	536. d	572. e	613. f
495. c	537. a,b	573. e	614. f
496. d	538. a	574. a-4, b-3	615. a
497. a	539. d	c-2,d-1	616. e
498. d	540. a	575. d	617. b
499. b	541. a	576. d	618. b
500. c	542. b	577. b	619. a
501. a	543. d	578. e	620. a
502. b	544. a	579. a	621. a-4, b-1
503. d	545. d	580. e	c-3,d-2
504. b	546. a	581. b	622. a-4, b-1
505. a	547. d	582. b	c-3,d-2
506. a	548. b	583. d	623. d
507. b	549. e	584. a	624. e
508. d	550. a	585. d	625. e
509. a	551. e	586. d	626. e
510. a	552. a	587. d	627. e
511. b	553. a	588. b,c,d	628. f
512. a	554. e	589. b	629. e
513.	555. a	590. d	630. d
514. b	556. d	591. a	631. a-4, b-1
515. b	557. c	592. d	c-3,d-2
516. b	558. a-4, b-1	593. d	632. a-4, b-1
517. d	c-3,d-2	594. a	c-3,d-2
518. d	559. a-4, b-3	595. d	633. f
519. d	c-2,d-1	596. e	634. a
520. d	560. e	597. e	635. e
521. d	561.	598. d	636. e
522. e	562. a,b	599. a	637. a
523. d	c,d	600. d	638. e
524. b	563. b	601. e	639. d
525. d	564. b	602 e	640. d
526. b	565. d	603. a	641. a,b
527. e	566. d	604. a	642. d
528. b	567. e	605. a	643. a
529. b	568. a	606. b	644. d
530. a	569. a-1	607. b	645. a

646.	d	687.	c	729.	b	768.	e
647.	d	688.	d	730.	b	769.	c,d
648.	d	689.	d	731.	b,c	770.	a
649.	b,c	690.	c	732.	a-4, b-1	771.	d
650.	a,b	691.	a		c-3,d-2	772.	d
651.	d	692.	c,kd	733.	a-4, b-1	773.	d
652.	a,b	693.	a		c-3,d-2	774.	d
653.	d	694.	d	734.	b,d	775.	a
654.	a-4, b-1	695.	d	735.	c	776.	e
	c-3,d-2	696.	b,c	736.	d	777.	b
655.	e	697.	d	737.	a	778.	a
656.	e	698.	c	738.	c	779.	a
657.	e	699.	d	739.	d	780.	d
658.	e	700	a	740.	a	781.	e
659.	b	701.	a	741.	a-4, b-1	782.	a
660.	c	702.	b		c-3,d-2	783.	a
661.	e	703.	d	742.	c	784.	a
662.	e	704.	d	743.	e	785.	e
663.	e	705.	c	744.	d	786.	e
664.	d	706.	d	745.	a,b	787.	b
665.	d	707.	a	746.	b	788.	a
666.	e	708.	b	747.	e	789.	c
667.	d	709.	a,b	748.	d	790.	c
668.	a	710.	a	749.	d	791.	b
669.	d	711.	b	750.	a	792.	d
670.	c	712.	a	751.	c	793.	c
671.	e	713.	a	752.	d	794.	c
672.	d	714.	b	753.	d	795.	c
673.	a	715.	c	754.	b	796.	a
674.	a,b	716.	d	755.	d	797.	a
675.	d	717.	d	756.	e	798.	a
676.	d	718.	a	757.	a	799.	b
677.	d	719.	d	758.	d	800.	a
678.	d	720.	a	759.	c,d	801.	e
679.	e	721.	a,b	760.	d	802.	a
680.	a	722.	d	761.	d	803.	e
681.	a,b	723.	c	762.	a	804.	e
682.	d	724.	a	763.	d	805.	d
683.	a,b,c	725.	a	764.	a	806.	d
684.	b	726.	b	765.	d	807.	a
685.	d	727.	a	766.	d	808.	a
686.	d	728.	b,c	767.	d	809.	d

810.	a	852.	d	893.	b	935.	e
811.	a,b	853.	c	894.	b	936.	a
812.	c	854.	e	895.	c	937.	b
813.	a	855.	d	896.	c	938.	a
814.	a	856.	e	897.	d	939.	a
815.	e	857.	e	898.	b	940.	a
816.	b	858.	a-4, b-1	899.	a	941.	b
817.	e		c-3,d-2	900.	a	942.	a
818.	c,d	859.	d	901.	a	943.	b
819.	d	860.	a	902.	a	944.	e
820.	d	861.	e	903.	d	945.	e
821.	d	862.	e	904.	c	946.	e
822.	d	863.	e	905.	d	947.	c,d
823.	a	864.	e	906.	c	948.	a,b
824.	b	865.	e	907.	a	949.	d
825.	b	866.	d	908.	a,b	950.	d
826.	a,b	867.	e	909.	e	951.	a
827.	a	868.	a	910.	a	952.	b
828.	c	869.	a,b	911.	e	953.	e
829.	d	870.	d	912.	a,b	954.	e
830.	a	871.	b	913.	e	955.	d
831.	a	872.	a	914.	e	956.	d
832.	a	873.	b	915.	a	957.	b
833.	e	874.	a	916.	b	958.	d
834.	a	875.	d	917.	a	959.	a
835.	b	876.	a	918.	a	960.	a
836.	a	877.	a	919.	a	961.	e
837.	a	878.	a	920.	b	962.	c,d
838.	d	879.	d	921.	a	963.	a
839.	e	880.	a	922.	d	964.	b
840.	d	881.	a	923.	e	965.	a
841.	b,c,d	882.	a	924.	e	966.	c
842.	c	883.	b	925.	a,b	967.	a
843.	d	884.	a	926.	a	968.	d
844.	d	885.	a,b	927.	a	969.	e
845.	b	886.	a	928.	e	970.	e
846.	e	887.	a	929.	b	971.	e
847.	a	888.	a	930.	c,d	972.	e
848.	d	889.	d	931.	e	973.	e
849.	a	890.	a	932.	a	974.	d
850.	e	891.	a	933.	d	975.	b
851.	e	892.	a	934.	d	976.	d

977.	a	1018.	e	1059.	a	1101.	a
978.	b	1019.	d	1060.	a	1102.	b,c,d
979.	b	1020.	c	1061.	a	1103.	e
980.	d	1021.	a,c	1062.	a	1104.	a
981.	a	1022.	a,b	1063.	a	1105.	c
982.	a	1023.	a,b	1064.	e	1106.	c
983.	a	1024.	a	1065.	e	1107.	e
984.	a	1025.	e	1066.	e	1108.	a,b
985.	c	1026.	c	1067.	a	1109.	a
986.	e	1027.	c	1068.	c	1110.	b
987.	a-4, b-1 c-3,d-2	1028.	e	1069.	d	1111.	d
988.	d	1029.	e	1070.	a	1112.	d
989.	c	1030.	d	1071.	c	1113.	d
990.	d	1031.	f	1072.	e	1114.	d
991.	e	1032.	d	1073.	a	1115.	e
992.	d	1033.	e	1074.	d	1116.	d
993.	d	1034.	e	1075.	a,c	1117.	d
994.	e	1035.	a-4, b-1 c-3,d-2	1076.	a	1118.	e
995.	a			1077.	e	1119.	a
996.	a	1036.	b	1078.	d	1120.	d
997.	e	1037.	d	1079.	b	1121.	c
998.	a	1038.	a,c	1080.	a	1122.	b
999.	d	1039.	a	1081.	d	1123.	a
1000.	c	1040.	d	1082.	a	1124.	a
1001.	e	1041.	a	1083.	c	1125.	a
1002.	c	1042.	a	1084.	e	1126.	b,c
1003.	e	1043.	d	1085.	b	1127.	e
1004.	e	1044.	d	1086.	d	1128.	a
1005.	e	1045.	a	1087.	c	1129.	d
1006.	c	1046.	b	1088.	e	1130.	a,b
1007.	d	1047.	d	1089.	c,d	1131.	d
1008.	a	1048.	e	1090.	e	1132.	d
1009.	a	1049.	e	1091.	d	1133.	d
1010.	e	1050.	a	1092.	e	1134.	c
1011.	d	1051.	a,b	1093.	e	1135.	d
1012.	a	1052.	b	1094.	d	1136.	e
1013.	e	1053.	a	1095.	b	1137.	d
1014.	b	1054.	a	1096.	e	1138.	a
1015.	a	1055.	b	1097.	a	1139.	e
1016.	a	1056.	a	1098.	e	1140.	e
1017.	,d	1057.	c	1099.	e	1141.	a,b,c
		1058.	d	1100.	b	1142.	d

1143.	a	1184.	e	1224.	e	1266.	d
1144.	a,b	1185.	e	1225.	d	1267.	a
1145.	e	1186.	d	1226.		1268.	a
1146.	e	1187.	a	1227.	a	1269.	b
1147.	a	1188.	a	1228.	e	1270.	a
1148.	d	1189.	a-4,	1229.	a	1271.	d
1149.	a		b-1 c-3,d-2	1230.	d	1272.	d
1150.	b	1190.	c	1231.	e	1273.	a
1151.	a	1191.	d	1232.	e	1274.	a-4,
1152.	a	1192.	a,b	1233.	b		b-1 c-3,d-2
1153.	e	1193.	d	1234.	e	1275.	a,b
1154.	e	1194.	e	1235.	e	1276.	d
1155.	c	1195.	d	1236.	a	1277.	d
1156.	e	1196.	d	1237.	d	1278.	c
1157.	e	1197.	c,d	1238.	a	1279.	e
1158.	d	1198.	c	1239.	c	1280.	d
1159.	e	1199.	e	1240.	e	1281.	d
1160.	e	1200.	a-4,	1241.	a	1282.	b,c
1161.	e		b-1 c-3,d-2	1242.	e	1283.	a,b
1162.	a	1201.	e	1243.	c	1284.	a,b,d
1163.	a,c	1202.	a	1244.	d	1285.	e
1164.	e	1203.	e	1245.	b	1286.	c
1165.	d	1204	e	1246.	e	1287.	b
1166.	a	1205.	b	1247.	a,b	1288.	e
1167.	e	1206.	a	1248.	d	1289.	b
1168.	d	1207.	a,b	1249.	a	1290.	d
1169.	e	1208.	c	1250.	e	1291.	d
1170.	d	1209.	e	1251.	d	1292.	b
1171.	d	1210.	e	1252.	a	1293.	b
1172.	e	1211.	d	1253.	a	1294.	a
1173.	a-4,	1212.	c	1254.	e	1295.	a
b-1 c-3,d-2		1213.	e	1255.	a	1296.	a
1174.	e	1214.	a	1256.	b	1297.	a
1175.	e	1215.	b	1257.	b	1298.	c
1176.	d	1216.	a	1258.	d	1299.	a
1177.	a	1217.	b	1259.	b	1300.	a
1178.	e	1218.	e	1260.	d		
1179.	e	1219.	c	1261.	e		
1180.	c	1220.	c	1262.	b		
1181.	a	1221.	d	1263.	b		
1182.	e	1222.	b	1264.	c,d		
1183.	e	1223.	a	1265.	c,d		

APPENDIX

MEDICINAL PLANTS.

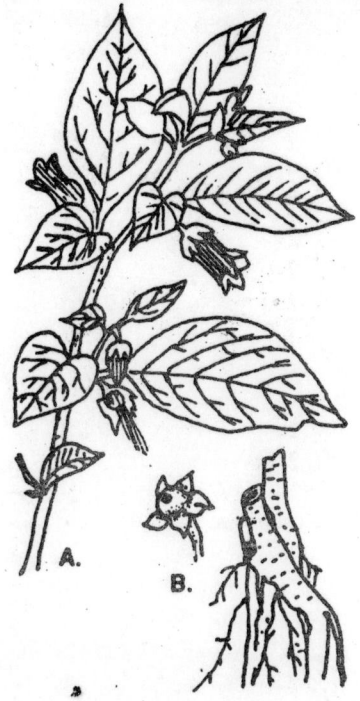

A.

B.

Fig. 1. *Atropa belladona* A. Plant; B. Fruit; and roots.

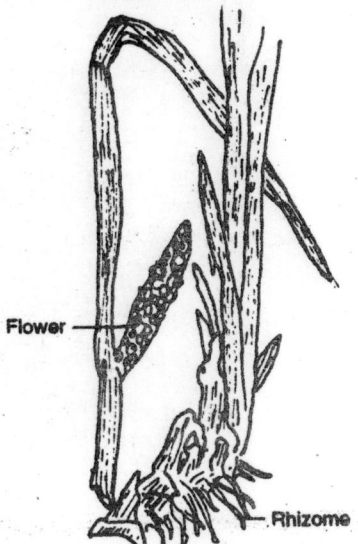

Flower

Rhizome

Fig. 2. *Acorus calamus* showing inflorescence and rhizome.

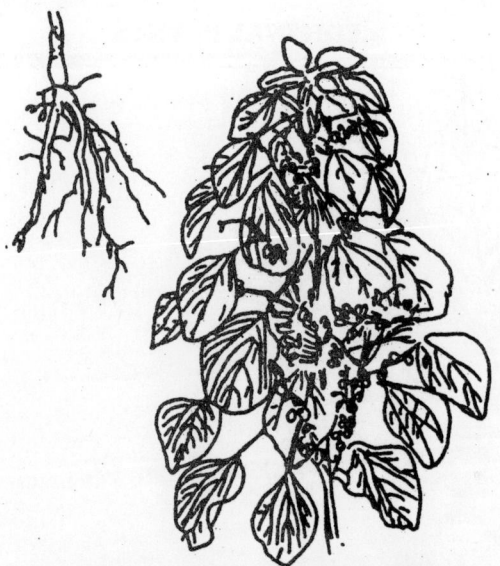

Fig. 3. Indian Acalypha (*Acalypha indica*).

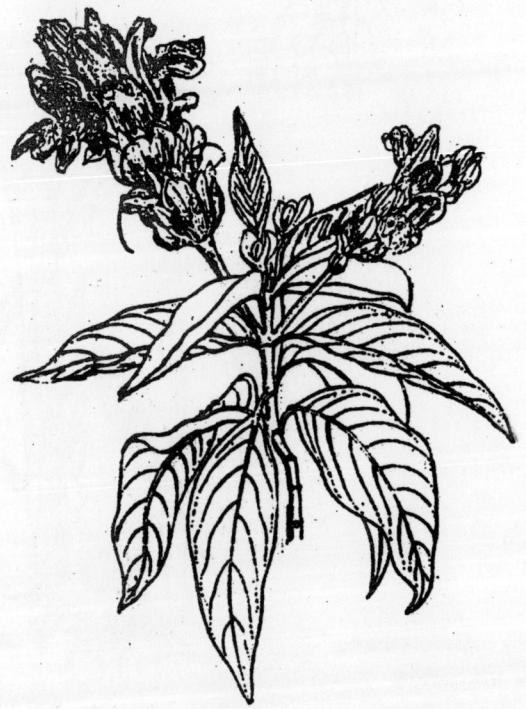

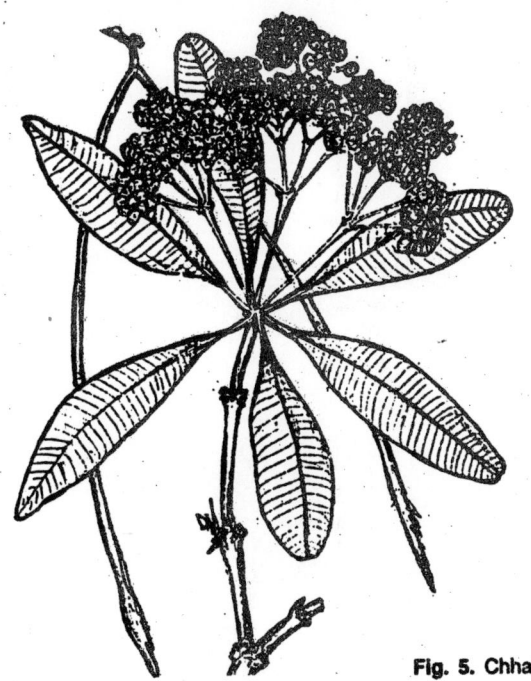

Fig. 5. Chhatim (*Alstonia scholaris*).

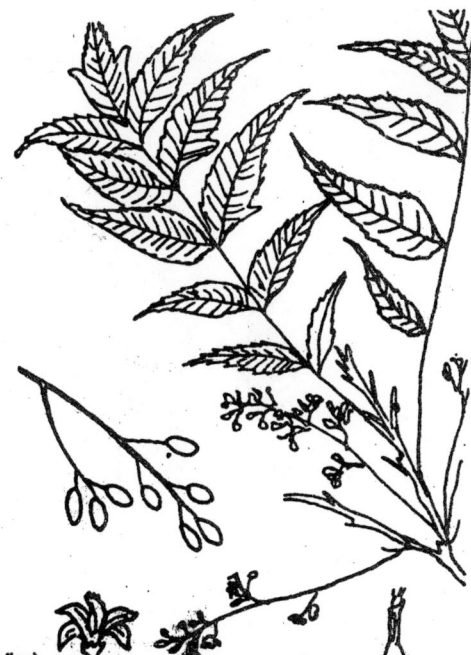

Fig. 6. Nim (*Azadirachta indica*).

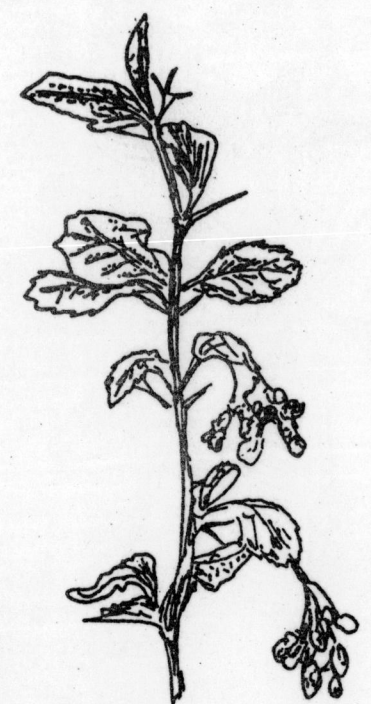

Fig. 7. Indian Barberry (*Berberis aristata*).

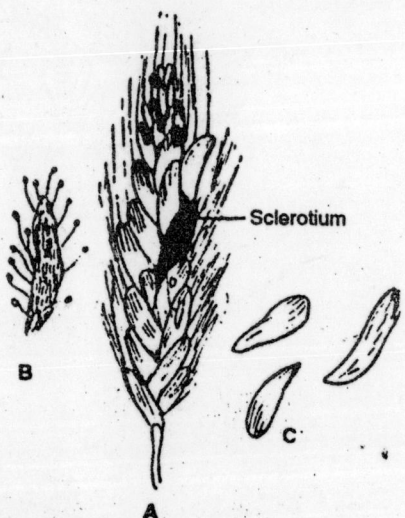

Fig. 8. *Claviceps purpurea* A. Infected spike; B. Sclerotium; C. Spores.

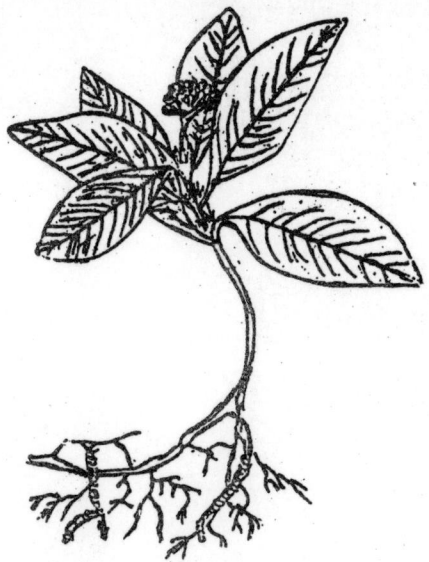

Fig. 9. *Cephaelis ipecacuanha*

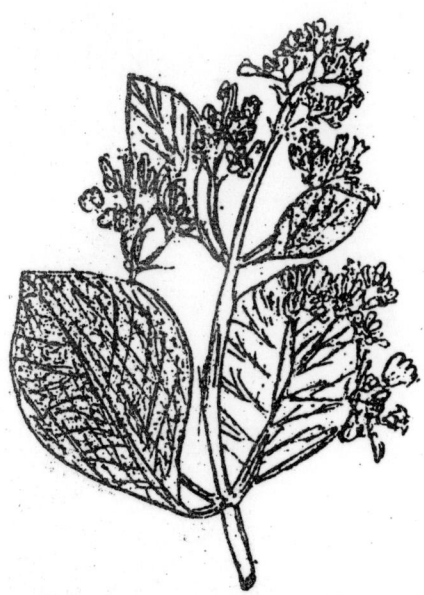

Fig. 10. *Cinchona (Calisaya).*

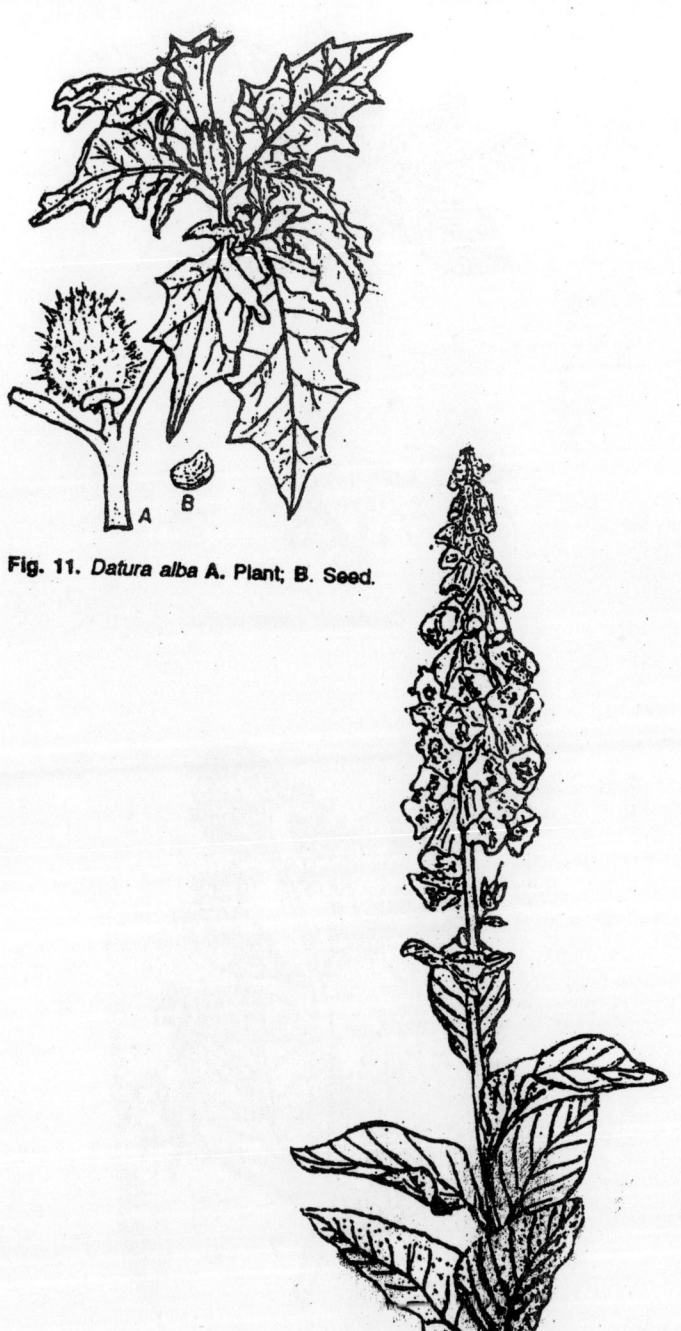

Fig. 11. *Datura alba* **A. Plant; B. Seed.**

Fig. 12. *Digitalis purpurea.*

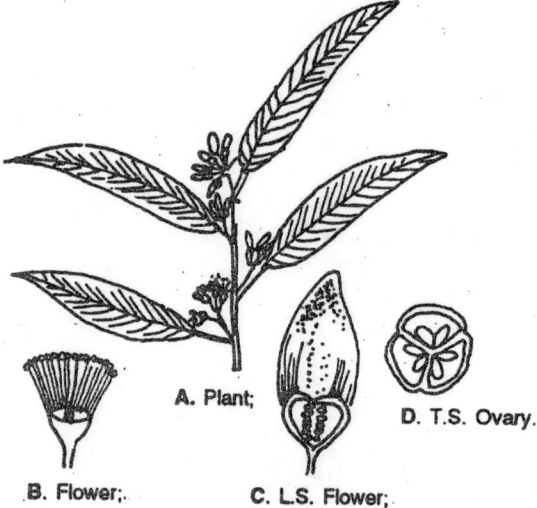

A. Plant;

B. Flower;

C. L.S. Flower;

D. T.S. Ovary.

Fig. 13. *Eucalyptus globulus.*

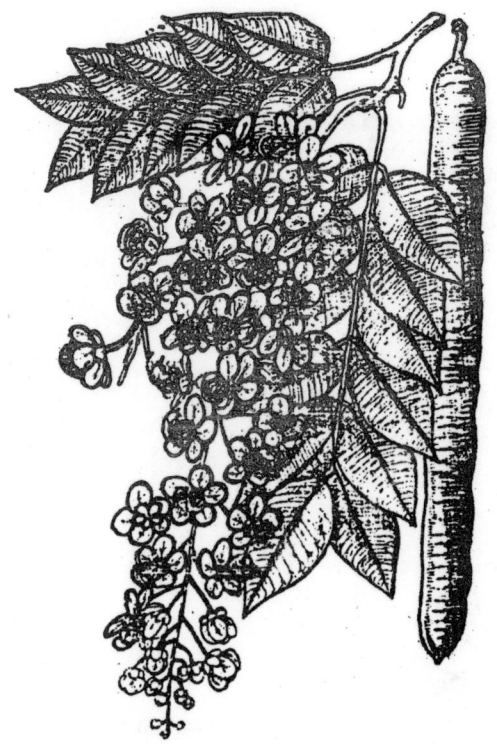

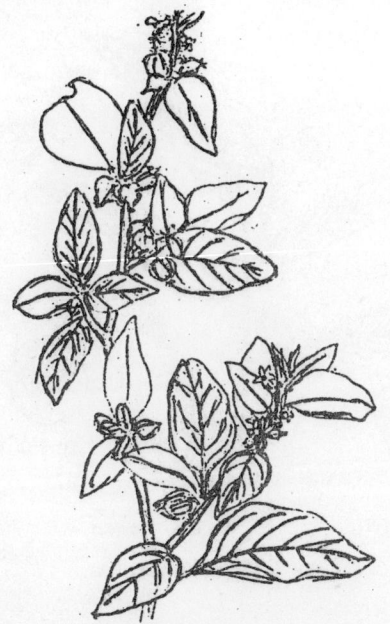

Fig. 15. Ashvagandha *(Withania somnifera).*

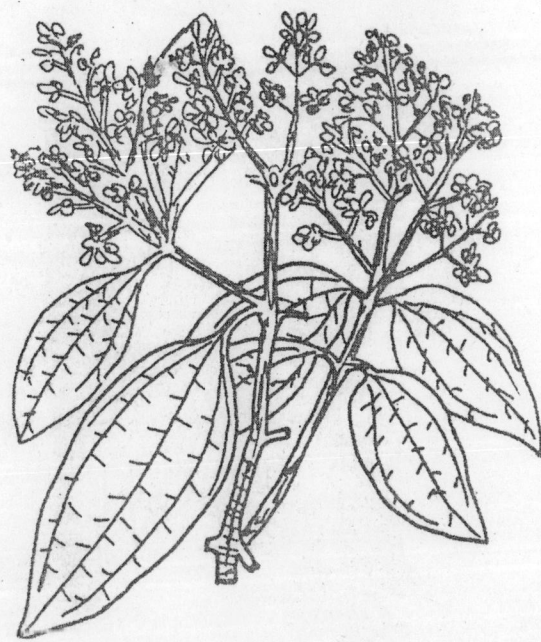

Fig. 16. Cinnamon *(Cinnamomum verum).*

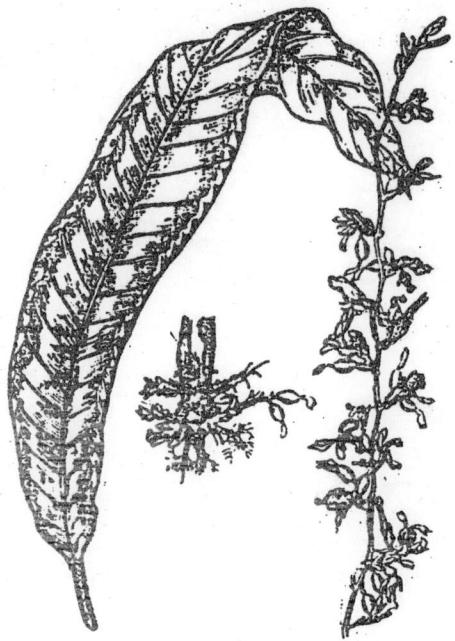

Fig. 17. Cardamom *(Elettaria cardamomum).*

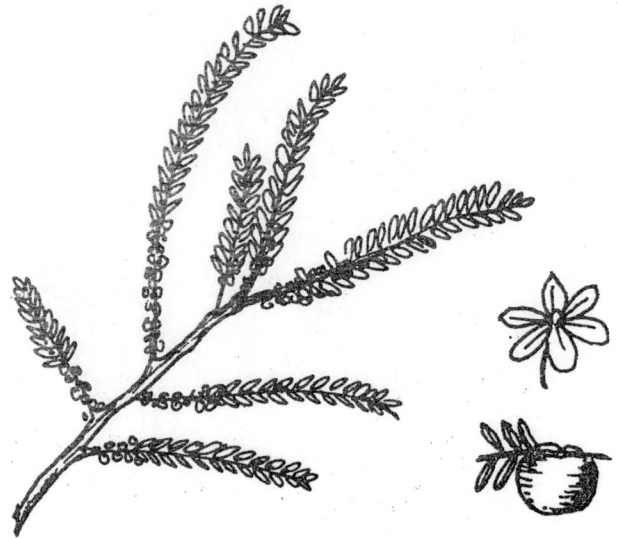

Fig. 18. Emblica *(Emblica officinalis).*

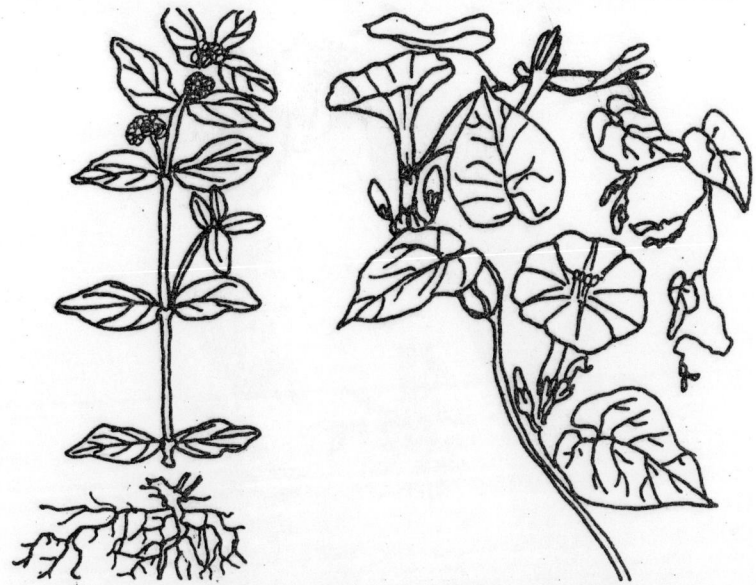

Fig. 19. Euphorbia *(Euphorbia hirta).*   **Fig. 20.** *Ipomoea purga.*

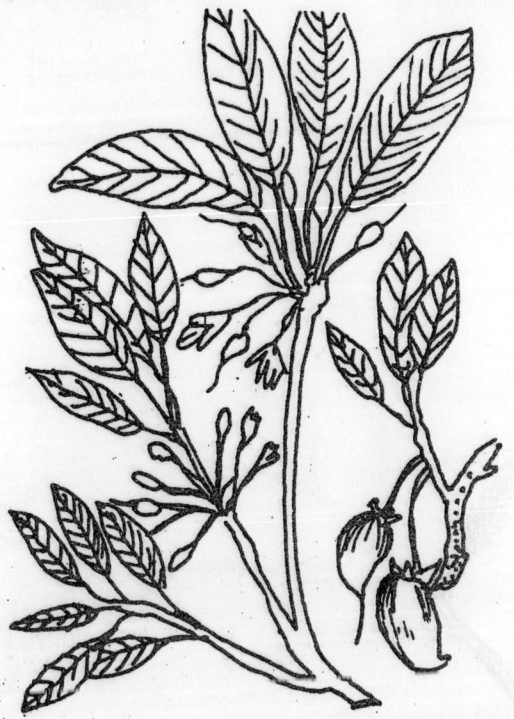

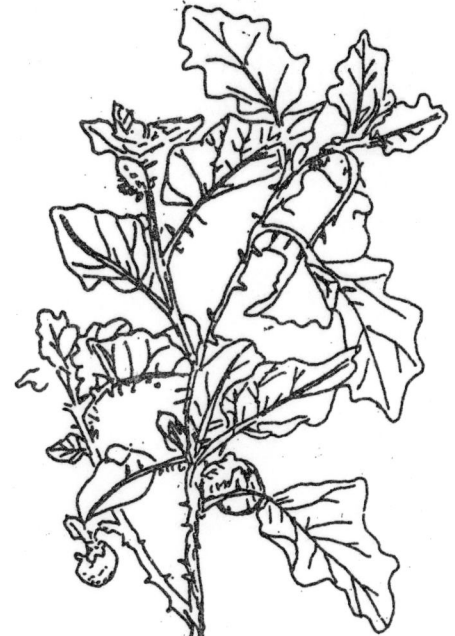

Fig. 22. Solanum *(Solanum incanum).*

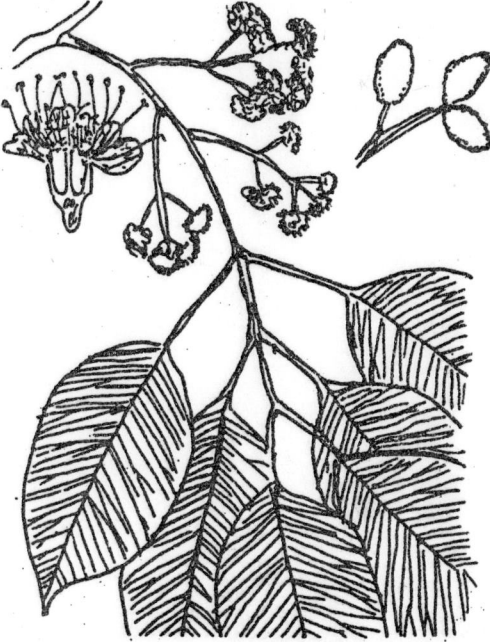

Fig. 23. Jambol *(Syzygium cumini).*

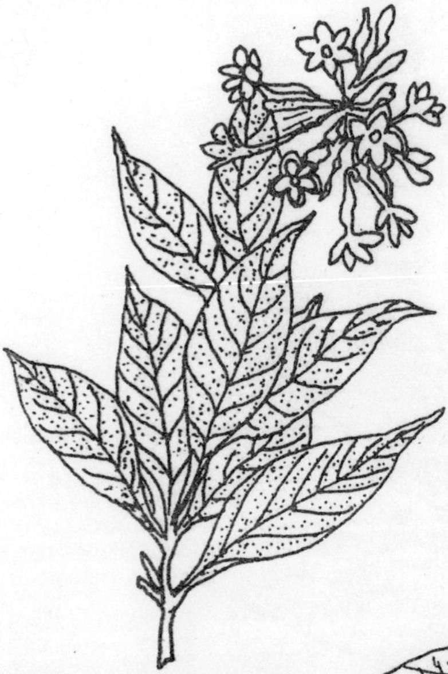

Fig. 24. *Rauvolfia serpentina.*
Plant.

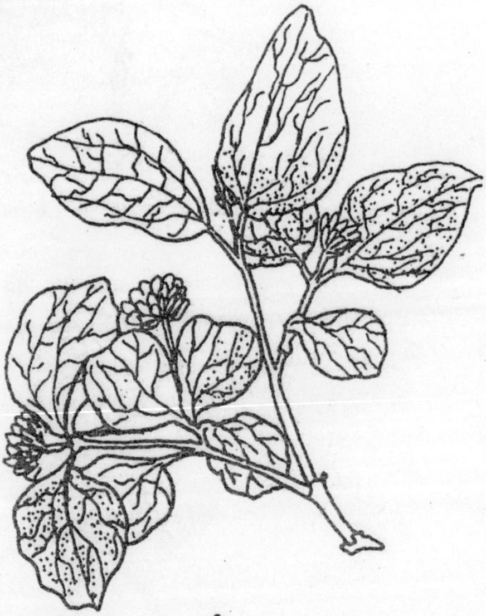

A

Fig. 25. Strychnos nux-vomica.

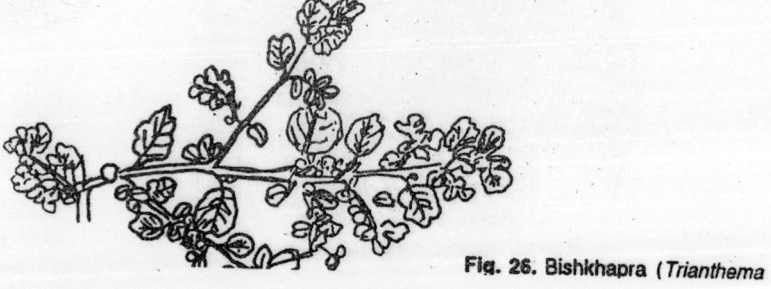

Fig. 26. Bishkhapra (*Trianthema*

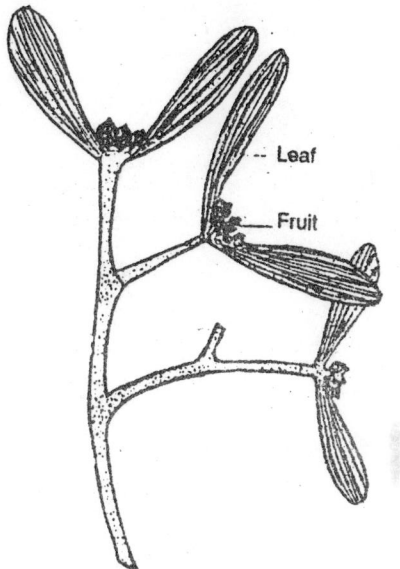

Fig. 27. *Viscum album* — Tv

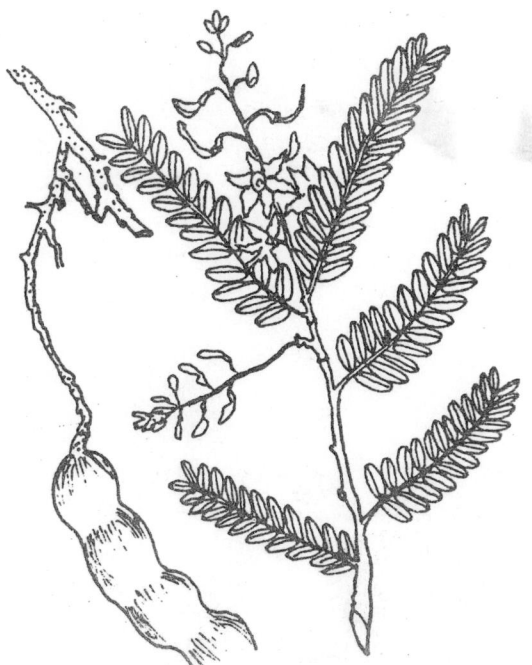

Fig. 28. Tamarind (*Tamarindus indica*).

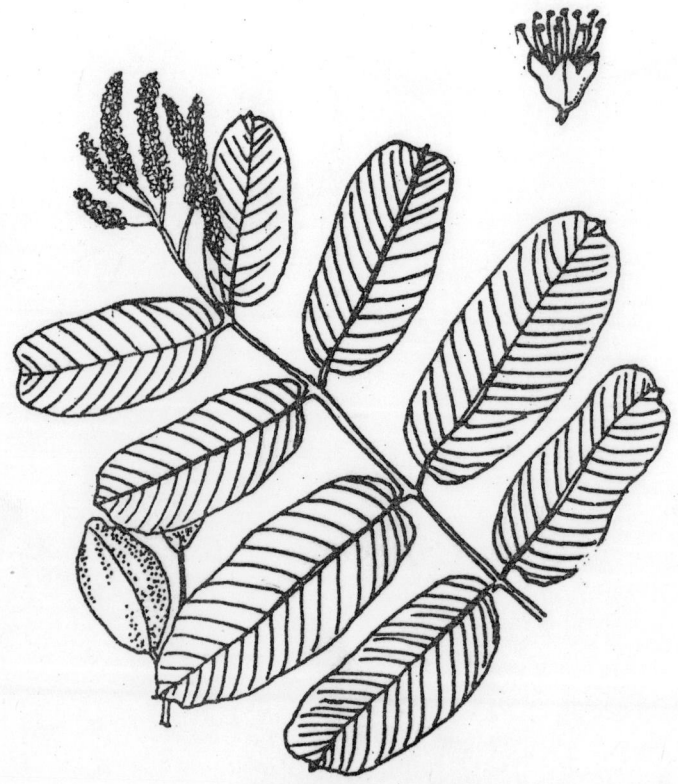

Fig. 29. Arjuna (*Terminalia arjuna*).

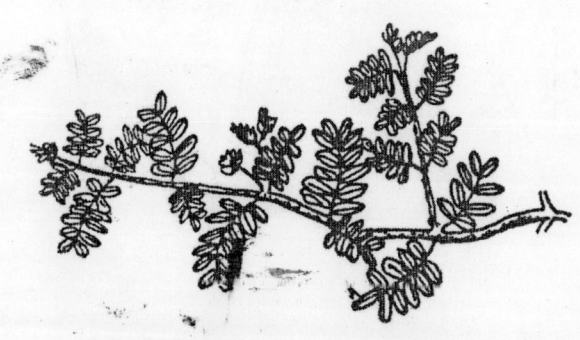

Fig. 30. Gokhru (*Tribulus terrestris*).